Members for Life

Richard Gerson, PhD
Gerson Goodson, Inc.

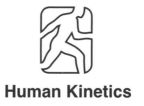

Human Kinetics

Library of Congress Cataloging-in-Publication Data

Gerson, Richard F.
    Members for life / by Richard Gerson.
       p.   cm.
    Includes index.
    ISBN 0-7360-0003-8
    1. Physical fitness centers--Customer services.   2. Relationship
marketing. I. Title.
    GV428.5.G49   1999
    613.7'068'--dc21   98-49538
                                                       CIP

ISBN: 0-7360-0003-8

Copyright © 1999 by Richard Gerson

Acquisitions Editor: Steven W. Pope, PhD; **Managing Editor:** Melinda Graham; **Copyeditor:** Heather Stith; **Proofreader:** Erin Cler; **Graphic Designer:** Jody Boles; **Graphic Artist:** Francine Hamerski; **Cover Designer:** Jack Davis; **Photographer (cover):** ©The Stock Market/Rob Lewine/1997; **Photographer (interior):** Tom Roberts; **Printer:** United Graphics

Printed in the United States of America   10 9 8 7 6 5 4 3 2 1

Human Kinetics
Web site: http://www.humankinetics.com/

United States: Human Kinetics, P.O. Box 5076, Champaign, IL 61825-5076
1-800-747-4457
e-mail: humank@hkusa.com

Canada: Human Kinetics, 475 Devonshire Road Unit 100, Windsor, ON N8Y 2L5
1-800-465-7301 (in Canada only)
e-mail: humank@hkcanada.com

Europe: Human Kinetics, P.O. Box IW14, Leeds LS16 6TR, United Kingdom
+44 (0) 113-278 1708
e-mail: humank@hkeurope.com

Australia: Human Kinetics, 57A Price Avenue, Lower Mitcham, South Australia 5062
(08) 82771555
e-mail: humank@hkaustralia.com

New Zealand: Human Kinetics, P.O. Box 105-231, Auckland Central
09-523-3462
e-mail: humank@hknewz.com

This book is dedicated with much love to my wife Robbie, and my sons Michael and Mitchell. They help me to understand the daily importance of a family being the ultimate reciprocal service organization. I love you all.

Contents

Acknowledgments   vi
Foreword   vii
Preface   viii
Introduction   xi

Part I Introduction to Customer Service and Member Retention   I

Chapter 1   The Importance of Customer Service to Health
            Club Success   3

Chapter 2   Making Customer Service Work for Your Members   19

Chapter 3   What Members Really Need, Want, and Expect   33

Chapter 4   Member Retention: The Backbone of Health
            Club Success   51

Part II Customer Service Skills   67

Chapter 5   The Telephone Is Your Member Service Lifeline   69

Chapter 6   The Service Recovery Process: Managing Angry
            Members and Complaining Members   83

Chapter 7   Three Critical Customer Service Skills: Building
            Rapport, Interpersonal Communication, and
            Effective Listening   99

Chapter 8   Measuring Member Satisfaction, Retention, and Loyalty 111

Chapter 9   Customer Service as a Powerful Marketing
            and Retention Tool   129

**Part III Member Relationship Management (Keeping
Members for Life)   145**

Chapter 10 The Member Relationship Management Process   147

Chapter 11 The Benefits of Retention and Loyalty   169

Part IV Techniques to Build Member Loyalty   187

Chapter 12 Member Retention Programs That Work   189

Appendix   50 Ways to Keep Your Members for Life   203

Index   213

About the Author   217

Acknowledgments

A book of this nature is never written alone. There are many people who have been involved in its development and production. I must first thank my clients in the health club and fitness industries who have allowed me to implement my ideas on customer service and member retention and show they work. John McCarthy and Janice DeGroot of the International Health, Racquet and Sportsclub Association (IHRSA), who have given me a forum for the last eight years to speak on these important topics, are also important to the development of this book. The people at Human Kinetics, who have been wonderful to me with this, my third book with HKP: Rainer Martens, Steve Pope, and Melinda Graham, I thank you so much.

And finally to my family. My wife Robbie, and my sons Michael and Mitchell. Thank you so much for putting up with my writing on our family trips, over the weekend, and late into the night. You are as much responsible for this book as I am.

Foreword

I know of no better way to highlight the value of Richard Gerson's newest book, *Members for Life*, than to specify exactly what you will find here:

- A customer service scorecard
- Customer service standards
- The 10 commandments of great customer service
- Fifteen ways to improve telephone customer service
- Twenty-five reasons members get upset
- Ten reasons why companies have poor customer service

These are but a few of the invaluable management tools that this book puts in the hands of club managers. Each one of these tools is a template against which you can examine your own personal and organizational service standards.

In these pages, you will find not only a compilation of everything Gerson has learned in the health club industry over the past 20 years, you'll also find new material that has not previously been part of his courses or seminars. For example, he has developed the first-ever typology of "difficult members," as well as specific guidelines for dealing effectively with them. He also has developed an original prototype for a different kind of club marketing plan that he calls the 10-step member-focused marketing plan. You'll never think about your marketing plan in the same way again. And Gerson presents his ideas in a clear and easy-to-read manner, providing sound advice. As he states, "*own* the telephone calls you take," "*beg* for member feedback," "do what works over and over again," "use members' names again, and again, and again," and "say thank you for every purchase, every referral, and *everything* else that a member does in your club."

In short, in *Members for Life* you will find groundbreaking material that will be of immediate benefit to you whether you're a novice or an experienced club manager. You're provided with the tool to think through your management and service opportunities from a fresh perspective. Gerson has been a conscientious student of the club industry for two decades, and he has saved his best ideas and writing for this superb text.

John McCarthy
Executive Director
IHRSA

Preface

So much is written today on the importance of customer service for success in general business. No business can succeed for any length of time without offering great customer service. Years ago, it seemed to be much easier to conduct business. You just made a product or service and sold it to the customer.

Then, something happened. Customers became more educated and more demanding of the company and people they bought from. They wanted more value for their money. They wanted to have their purchase risks reduced so that, if something went wrong with the purchase, they could return or exchange it. They wanted to be treated with respect by the salespeople. In short, they refused to be pushed around any more by business. They wanted better customer service.

The same thing happened in the health club industry. Fifteen years ago, someone would buy a lifetime membership to a club and, quite often, pay it off in full. Then, if that club went out of business in a year or two (maybe three or four), the member would lose all the money that was paid in. As it turned out, lifetime memberships meant the lifetime of the club, not the lifetime of the member.

Without any recourse, these former members were burned, so they started screaming for better service and more of a guarantee. A three-day cooling off period was established and enforced. This period gives a person who purchases a membership 72 hours after that to decide whether to keep the membership or receive a full refund. Although this made members feel a little better, because it reduced some of their risks of purchasing a membership, it still did not provide the level of service they were looking for.

When members got into the club, they were treated like numbers or bodies, rather than people. All the promises that were made during sales presentations never appeared. Promises such as personal attention, personalized programs, constant supervision, no wait for machines, and no overcrowded classes became just so much rhetoric. The clubs promised these things but could not deliver. In today's customer service lingo, they overpromised and underdelivered, which is as good as signing your own death warrant.

What did these service miscues mean for the visionary club owner? For those who saw the light early on, it was the opening of a treasure chest of opportunities. Although some clubs couldn't change their policies and procedures quickly to accommodate members, perhaps because they were part of a larger chain, other clubs could immediately begin giving customers what they wanted. Member service began to be a key differentiating factor in selling memberships; service also leveled the playing field so all sizes of clubs could compete.

Today, it seems as though all clubs promote superior quality and high levels of customer service. Yet not everyone delivers on these promises. Talking the talk is no longer enough. Again, customers are too smart. You must walk the walk. Otherwise, members will walk away from your club and go somewhere else.

Every club is capable of providing superior customer service and distinguishing themselves from the competition in some service-related manner. Because almost all clubs today have similar equipment, training programs, and qualified staff, member service and what I call member relationship management (MRM) may be the only differentiating factors left in the entire health club industry. It's just a matter of knowing how important customer service and the MRM process is to the success of your club.

In my previous books on marketing in the health and fitness industry, I suggested that every club can remain profitable regardless of economic conditions if they applied the marketing strategies and tactics I described in those books. Now, I'm taking that bold statement a step further. When you provide great customer service to your members, you will survive no matter what happens to the economy or who comes into the neighborhood as competition. People will do business with people they like, and we all like people who provide us with courteous and friendly service. Members who are treated well will remain loyal to the clubs that take care of them.

That's what this book is all about. It shows club owners, regardless of their club's size, how to implement customer service and MRM systems that are user-friendly and results-oriented. The book also describes how to use customer service as a powerful marketing tool to attract and retain members. You'll also learn how to measure the quality of your service along with your members' levels of satisfaction, retention, and loyalty. Then this book does something few, if any, of the other customer service books on the market do: it talks about the importance of customer service and member retention in health clubs from a business perspective.

Many articles have been published in many of the trade magazines about the importance of customer service and member retention. Although some of these articles focus on the business side of service and retention, many of them view these two important business issues as merely programs to be implemented. Programs are helpful, but these issues are greater than a member retention program of the month.

Success in today's club industry is dependent on great customer service for members and a systematic process that engages everyone in the club in building and managing member relationships. To date, only a handful of magazine articles and presentations at conventions have addressed these important issues, and that is why this book was written. This book teaches you exactly how to develop the most important customer service skills you and your staff will need to dazzle and delight your members.

The book begins by focusing on the importance of customer service to your members, what members really need, want, and expect from your club, and why member retention and loyalty are important to the success of your club business. The middle part of the book focuses on the skills you need to handle the telephone properly, to improve your listening and communication skills that are so important to service success, to manage, serve, and satisfy angry or complaining members and turn them into future sales, and to use customer service as a marketing tool. Finally, and just as importantly, the last part of the book covers a wide variety of techniques you can use to retain your members, to manage the member relationship and life cycle process, and to build members' loyalty and commitment in order to keep members for life.

Customer service is critical to the success of every club. You can have great marketing that brings in the members for the first purchase, but it's going to be your level of service that keeps them coming back year after year. Every customer deserves a level of service that is 10 times the amount of each purchase they're making. When you do this, you ensure their commitment and loyalty to your club business. When you don't do this, your members become somebody else's members. And as you'll learn in this book, the more times a member renews with you or makes repeat purchases in your pro shop or restaurant, the more profitable that member becomes to you.

So in order to keep members from "voting with their feet," club owners must establish and implement customer service systems and member relationship management programs that are designed to help gain, retain, and keep members for life. This book provides the blueprint for that journey. You must do more than read it. You must use it on a daily basis as a guide for owning and operating a club, and as a training manual for your staff. Then you can be sure your club will successfully serve and satisfy its members and keep them for life.

Introduction
Techniques to Build Member Loyalty

Throughout this book, you'll read about many different ways you can increase member retention and build loyalty. You should already know that retention and loyalty are the keys to your future success. I'm going to give you a few specific suggestions to increase the loyalty of your members.

Begin by remembering that you must create a psychological bond with your members. They must become interdependent with you and feel committed to you. Both of you must work together to help each other achieve your goals. Members want to get fit; you want to run a successful club. What can you do to make members want to stay in a long-term relationship with you and your club? If you answered, "Love the members," you're right. Although you won't love the members in the same way that you love your spouse or children, you still must love your members. Show members you care. Tell them you care. Make sure they know you care about them.

Here are some other things you can do to quickly build member loyalty.

• **Create a service-oriented culture.** The focus of everything in your club must be on service. There must be total commitment from the owners and managers to this service concept, and everyone must support the line staff in their efforts to serve the members. Post your service commitments and philosophies in a conspicuous place. Celebrate your service accomplishments by rewarding employees for excellent service performance. Work with the members to learn what they need and want from you and give it to them. Believe that service is more important than sales, and your sales will increase.

• **Empower employees to serve.** Saying you want to provide great service in order to retain members is not enough. You must give your staff the latitude and leeway to do whatever they deem necessary to take care of the members.

Empower them, give them responsibility, and then hold them accountable for their service performances. The two worst things you can do are to tell your employees they are empowered and then have them check with you for an answer to every member situation. The other thing is to hold them accountable for service delivery but not give them the authority to serve. These actions send mixed messages and confuse the staff and the members. Empowerment is a two-way street where staff gets to serve and management must trust. If you need to, begin the empowerment process by identifying boundaries for your staff and then letting them expand those boundaries based on performance.

• **Reward member loyalty.** Set up programs that reinforce good member behavior. Establish and publicize your reward program. Celebrate those members who are loyal. The longer a person stays with you, the more you should reinforce that positive behavior.

• **Beg for member feedback.** The more you get your members involved in the operations of your club (in an advisory role), the longer they will stay with you. Everyone loves to have their opinion solicited, and they like it even more when you implement their suggestions. Get member feedback in every way possible. Use surveys, focus groups, informal discussions, advisory councils, and anything else you can think of. Don't just talk about the importance of member feedback. Go out and get it.

• **Align values.** Find out the things your members value the most. Align your business values to their personal and business values. When they see how much in agreement you are with the way they live their lives, they will stay with you longer. This is another way to cement the psychological bond between you and your members.

• **Deliver on your promises.** When you promise something to a member, you are making a guarantee that you will keep your promise. For many years, we were told to underpromise and overdeliver. Today, members are too smart to fall for that. They know when you're intentionally lowering their expectations so you can meet certain performance levels. You must make your performance promises and guarantees at a level that meets the members' expectations and deliver on those promises. That's the only way you'll get them to keep coming back and stay loyal.

• **Use high-touch, support it with high-tech.** Although computers and technology are essential to your success, using a high-touch approach is even more important when building member loyalty. People have to know you care about them. Keep in contact with your members. Literally touch them. Let them know you're there for them and that you care about them. Once you've done this, you can support your personal efforts with your database marketing and customer service.

• **Know who your right customers are.** Right customers are the members who are the most profitable and who place the least strain and drain on your service delivery. They join, they buy products, they use the facility, they make referrals, and they are happy. You can identify your right members by profiling those members who are already with you for the long term. Then you use your marketing, sales, and service efforts to go after other right members.

• **Make members feel important.** People love when other people pay attention to them. You need to treat every member like a VIP. Make members feel special and important. Go out of your way to make their day. They will then go out of their way to make yours.

• **Be accessible to members.** This statement goes for you personally and your hours of operation. Be open and available to meet with members and talk with them when it's convenient for them. Accessibility is a major determining factor in whether a customer stays with a supplier. In this case, it will determine whether a member stays with your club or joins another one.

• **Maintain your commitments.** If you schedule an appointment with a member, or promise to call a member at a certain time, or promise to do something for a member, keep your commitments. No excuses. Just keep them, and the members will come to rely on you. Your dependability and integrity will go a long way toward motivating the members to stay with you.

• **Develop and implement motivational retention programs.** I will tell you throughout the book that retention is a business proposition for you, not just a program of the month. However, you must realize that your retention programming can be very motivational and financially rewarding when it is done right. Chapter 12 will discuss 25 retention programs that work in our industry. Make sure your retention programming fits in with your service efforts, your retention approach to business, and your loyalty-building campaign.

• **Anticipate changes in member needs.** Stay one step ahead of your members. If you get to know them as well as possible, you can anticipate what they will need from you next. Have it ready to provide for them. This readiness will provide them with a wow factor and will dazzle and delight them; they will reward you by staying with you.

• **Do what works over again, only better.** Take a look at what you've accomplished. Analyze why it worked so well. Then figure out how you can improve on any of your loyalty-building techniques. Implement the improved techniques and watch your club business grow.

part one

Introduction to Customer Service and Member Retention

CHAPTER 1

The Importance of Customer Service to Health Club Success

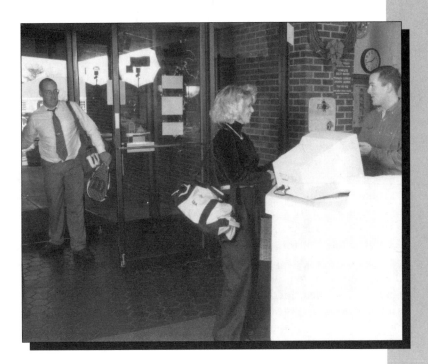

C ustomer service is the critical factor for succeeding in the health club business today. You must provide customer service that is far superior to that offered by your competitors in order for your health club to attract and keep members who remain loyal and help you make a profit. Although you may be in this business to help people improve their health and fitness levels, you must always remember that you're still in a business. Therefore, to remain in business, you must make a profit by effectively servicing your members.

One fitness center that I worked with began conducting member service and satisfaction surveys. They wanted to find out exactly how the members felt about the treatment they were receiving from the staff. Some of the questions on the survey were related to the time of day the member used the facility. When we analyzed the results of the survey, we found that the morning members were much more satisfied than the afternoon or evening members.

So we investigated further. We learned that the front desk receptionist in the morning took the time to learn the names of each and every member who regularly came in. She welcomed them by name with a bright and cheery "Good morning" every day. The afternoon and evening receptionists were more concerned with completing their job requirements properly, which consisted of swiping the member's card so the attendance data would be automatically entered into the computer. The morning receptionist also did this task, but only after she had greeted the member and made sure the member entered the facility smiling and with a positive impression. After we trained the afternoon and evening receptionists to provide the high level of friendly service that their morning colleague offered, the next survey showed dramatic improvements in everyone's satisfaction levels.

So what does this example tell us? Something as simple as greeting the members by name and using a positive, uplifting tone of voice goes a long way toward setting the tone for superior member service. If we would have looked at the membership renewal rates, you can bet that the morning members would have renewed at a greater rate than the afternoon or evening members because of the great customer service they received.

A high level of customer service leads to increased retention, lower acquisition costs, and higher profitability. Just like in the general business world, where customer retention and lower customer acquisition costs determine the success of a business, member retention and lowered member acquisition costs result in the greatest profit for health clubs. Profitability is not determined by the highest cost per membership or the number of memberships sold, as many club owners and managers mistakenly believe. These numbers only affect cash flow, and cash flow does not always translate into profits; just ask any entrepreneur. Profits are based on members spending more within your club than you have to spend to get them there, which is a function of the service you provide. That's why, throughout the book, I link superior service, member retention, and member loyalty with profitability.

You've probably read and heard a great deal about the importance of customer service and how clubs should treat their members. If you've attended any of my industry presentations, or read any of my magazine articles on the subject or my other books, or are a reader of industry publications such as *CBI*, *Club Industry*, and *Fitness Management*, to name a few, then you know this topic is always in vogue. Yet despite all the books, articles, audiotapes, and videos on customer service and member retention, thousands of clubs and other fitness-related businesses still have not gotten the message. That's very unfortunate, because it's an easy message to get.

Common Sense Customer Service

Much of customer service comes down to simple common sense. What do I mean by common sense customer service? It's everything you and your employees do to satisfy members. That means you give them what they want and make sure they're happy. If you just manage complaints, offer refunds, or smile at members, you are only providing a small part of excellent customer service. Customer service also means going out of your way for the customer, doing everything possible to satisfy the customer, and making decisions that benefit the customer, sometimes even at the expense of the business. (When this situation occurs, consider the future potential of that customer's business with you. We'll discuss this issue more later when I cover the lifetime value of a member.)

Now don't believe for a minute that I am saying you should give away the store to the member. I am saying you must know when and how often the member/customer is right and when it is worth your while to provide extra service to satisfy that member. You've probably heard that the customer is always right. Well, that's not exactly true. Sometimes customers are wrong, as when they try to take advantage of you

> **While not always right, the customer is always the customer.**

or they become disruptive or abusive. Then they definitely are not right. Although they may not always be right, they are always customers; that's the only point you have to remember.

With this new view of the customer in mind, you and your staff must make all your service decisions based on the situation, what the member wants, and how it affects your business. Treat every member as an individual and as he or she wants to be treated with respect to the situation that member is in. Interact with the member as a person, not as a number on a membership card or in your database. You must also treat every service situation as unique. Don't let inflexible rules, regulations, policies, and procedures stop you from making your members happy. Just use good old common sense.

The Importance of Customer Service

How important is customer service to the success of your club business? It can make or break you. You and your competitors are selling the same product or

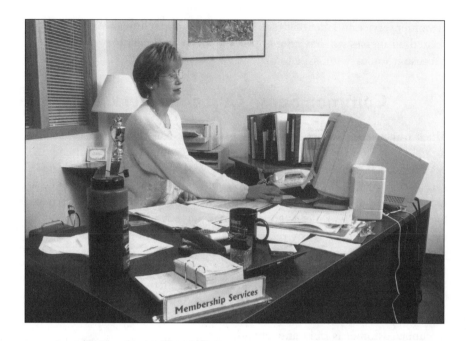

service (memberships) at basically the same price. You really have nothing within the product or service to differentiate you from them. You all have similar cardiovascular equipment, free weights, strength training equipment, lockers, showers, and so on. You both are located within the potential member's driving/living/working area. Both of the clubs are clean and bright. Under these circumstances, what makes members buy from you instead of your competitors?

Could it be the way you and your employees treat members? How about the way you answer the telephone, or listen to their requests for information on the memberships you're selling? What about the appearance of your club? What about the additional service you provide after the sale? Do you treat members as part of your family, or do they just become numbers after they join? Do you involve them in activities with your staff and other members? What else do you do to make them feel special? All these things relate to customer service and the impression members have of you. If these impressions and perceptions are positive, members not only will do business with you one time, they will do business with you repeatedly. If these perceptions are negative, or if you have done something to upset a customer, you can be sure he or she will go down the street to one of your competitors.

Think about the last time you had poor service, either at a restaurant, an airport, a retail store, or another health club. Remember what you thought and how you felt. Did you have anything nice to say about the place? Would you refer friends and family to that place after its employees treated you badly? I don't think so. Why would you want your members to experience any of those negative or painful feelings? You know how you perceived the poor service situation and what you planned to do about it. You decided to take your business elsewhere; don't you think your members will do the same?

As you'll see in the following pages, many of your members will not complain. They'll just vote with their feet. But there are things you can do to prevent them from walking out, which is what the rest of this book is about. Remember that your goal in providing great customer service is to create members for life.

The Payoff of Superior Customer Service

Several years ago, you couldn't pay some clubs to train their employees to provide good customer service. Either the clubs did not view customer service as important, or they didn't think the training was important, or they didn't think the employees warranted training beyond specific job skills. Some clubs I've worked with in the past actually felt that members would come in, buy a membership, use the club, and eventually leave anyway, so it didn't matter whether you were nice to them. Many businesses have this same incorrect attitude with regard to their customers. Can you believe that in light of today's competitive environment?

Although there may have been a time when people would just accept how you treated them and continue to do business with you, that is no longer the case. People are more educated, and they demand more for their dollar. If you don't provide them with great customer service, they will just find someone else who will.

About 20 years ago, when racquetball was beginning to boom as a club sport, I became a pretty good player. I was good enough to compete at the open level in tournaments and to teach racquetball at various clubs, so I had several local fitness and racquetball clubs competing for my membership. They made all sorts of promises about how much I could use the facility, how often I could play, the availability of fitness equipment, how my wife would be treated, and so on.

During a two-year period, I represented three different clubs because they did not live up to their service promises. They said one thing, and then delivered another, so I left. And I cost them more than my own and my wife's membership. I took all my referrals with me, plus all the private lessons. Not to mention that I came back and beat their representatives in the racquetball tournaments. So they suffered financial loss as well as psychological loss, or at least a decrease in their industry image.

> **Customer service always pays off.**

I tell you this personal story not to show off, but to illustrate an important point about customer and member service. Customer service pays. It really does not cost you anything. Yes, you may have to spend some dollars up front in training programs for your staff, and you may have to give away some things that you normally wouldn't in order to keep a member happy. Plus, revamping or revising your service delivery systems and processes within your club usually involves some other costs. But in the long run, customer service always pays off.

The way it pays off the most is in long-term customer or member retention. Keeping members and doing business with them repeatedly is much less expensive and much more profitable than trying to find new members all the time. Keep in mind that it costs you much more to acquire a new member than it does to retain a current member. To get a new member, you must factor in marketing, advertising, and selling costs. To do business with a current member, you must consider the cost of communicating with that person regularly.

Some Examples of the Dollar Value of Customer Service

Some clubs know the cost of acquiring a new member; others do not have a clue what new member acquisition costs them. Those clubs that know what it costs to acquire a member are bending over backward to keep the members they have happy. As for the others, many club owners unfortunately are not even aware of the extraordinary costs of losing a customer. They just figure that if someone stops doing business with them one day (lets a membership lapse), another person will join. Wrong!

There are three things you must know about the payoff for providing excellent customer service. First, acquiring a new member costs five to six times more than conducting business with a current or former member does. Suppose you calculate that the cost of acquiring a new member is $500, and you figure out that it costs you only about $100 to do business with a current member. That $400 savings becomes your club's profit. (Some research estimates say getting a new customer/member costs 10 times more than conducting business with a current one does. What does this new figure do for your profit margins?)

Second, whenever you lose a customer, there are costs associated with replacing that customer along with the loss of revenue that customer's membership would have provided during the replacement period. There is also something called lost opportunity revenue, which is all the potential money you could have made from the member if you kept her or him loyal and that person continued to purchase from you over an extended period of time.

The third thing is the cost of negative word of mouth. Whenever you lose a member, it is usually due to a bad experience that person had with you. You can control between 96 percent and 99 percent of the reasons people stop doing business with you, depending on the type of club you have, so you should only lose a small number of members. But if you dissatisfy even one member, that person may tell up to 20 people about the bad service they received. The odds are that these 20 people will not do business with you at all. Calculate that lost opportunity revenue over a 3-, 5-, or 10-year period. If that's not mind-boggling enough, consider the geometric progression of 20 people telling 20 people who tell another 20 people not to join your club because you provide bad service.

Add the costs of these three reasons together, and you get a pretty good idea of how valuable and profitable providing superior customer service is and how very costly providing poor service is. With these costs in mind, the question is not whether you can afford to train your staff to provide excellent customer service; it's can you afford not to? Consider the payoff in money earned or saved by keeping your members against what it costs you to replace them. Combine replacement costs with the money you are losing because a dissatisfied customer's friends, who would have joined your club, now will have nothing to do with you because of the way you treated their friend, your former member. To put it simply, customer service and long-term customer satisfaction and retention are vitally important to your success in the club business.

Quality Customer Service Is Profitable

High-quality customer service is as much a marketing tool for your business as it is a management approach or philosophy. Service quality improves your marketing because it motivates members to tell others about you, and these referrals essentially create a customer sales force. Remember, the least expensive way to acquire new members is through word-of-mouth referrals. What better way is there to get new members than to have their friends tell them to do business with you? Isn't that why all clubs conduct "Member-Get-A-Member" promotions as well as other membership promotions? We'll talk more about this concept later in the book. For now, let's agree that providing superior customer service is very profitable.

> *Customers are the life-blood of a business.*

Good service also improves club management and makes it easier because everybody is committed to satisfying the customer. Employees are happier knowing that they can do whatever it takes, without fear of reprisal or repercussions, to satisfy the customer. The results are increased satisfaction and referrals on the part of the customer, increased productivity from the employees, and increased profitability for the business because everyone is working toward the same goal: member satisfaction and retention.

Now that you know how important great customer service is to your success in business, let's get to the heart of the matter: money. The next section will provide you with what I call "Startling Service Statistics" gathered from a variety of research sources. Then comes a formula for calculating the costs of poor service and relating that to member acquisition and retention. Finally, I provide you with information on a little-known, yet vitally important, service-related, marketing concept combination called lifetime value and marginal net worth of a member. If this information and your own calculations don't motivate you to provide the ultimate in customer service, then maybe you should think about what you'll be doing when your competitors steal your members from you.

Startling Service Statistics

Remember that these statistics have been compiled from a variety of sources over the last 10 years. You might have seen, heard, or read about some of these figures already, as well as some other numbers that are different from those presented here. The important point is that these statistics and numbers are designed to educate and inform you about the importance of customer service. If, for any reason, your club's numbers don't correspond with the ones presented here, call me personally, and we'll discuss how these numbers relate to your business.

• Only 4 percent of your members will complain. That means that you never hear from 96 percent of your members who may have a problem. To make matters worse, 91 percent of those who do have a problem or a complaint will just leave your club because they feel that complaining will not do any good. That's why you must solicit complaints so you can get feedback, make changes, and continue to do business with the complainers. In fact, complainers are more likely to stay with you after you resolve their problems than noncomplainers are.

• For every complaint you receive in your club, there are 26 other members with unresolved problems or related complaints. Six of those 26 members have major or severe complaints. You need to set up a system to get these people to communicate with you. They are your best source of information to improve your club operations.

• When you quickly resolve complaints to the satisfaction of the member, 54 to 70 percent of these members will continue to stay with you. They'll renew their memberships, buy from your pro shop, and join your ancillary programs. The quicker you resolve their complaints, the greater the percentage of repeat business. Up to 95 percent of your complaining members will buy from you again when they are quickly and completely satisfied.

• It costs five to six times more to get a new member than it does to get a current member to renew, repurchase, or refer. It also costs less to get lapsed members to rejoin than to it does to acquire new members. Factor in lifetime value and marginal net worth calculations, and you'll understand why it is more profitable to do business with current customers than to recruit new ones.

• Dissatisfied members will tell up to 10 other people about their dissatisfaction, and 13 percent of those dissatisfied members will tell up to 20 people. This negative word of mouth can kill you, so you must make sure your club is working for its members.

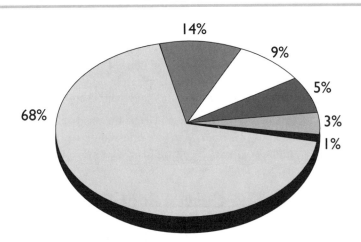

Members stop doing business with you for the following reasons:

■ 1 percent die

■ 3 percent move away

■ 5 percent look for other club relationships

■ 9 percent start working out at other clubs

■ 14 percent are dissatisfied with your service or the club product you offer

■ 68 percent don't like the way they were treated by your staff

These percentages reveal an exciting possibility within their apparent negativity. Depending on the type, size, and scope of your club, you can control up to 99 percent of the reasons a member would stop coming to your facility. That's why member service and retention programs are so important to your success in the club industry. If you don't use these programs, it's going to cost you big time.

FIGURE 1.1 *Why members stop doing business with you*

• Satisfied members, on the other hand, tell only between three and five people about their positive experiences with your club. This means that you may have to work up to five times as hard to satisfy enough members to counteract the negative potential of one dissatisfied member. That's why member retention processes, programs, and systems are so important.

• When your club provides superior service, you can realize an increase of between 6 percent and 10 percent in market share. People will want to join your club because of the great service you provide. Plus, you can charge more for better service, increase your market share and profit margins, and lower your acquisition costs because of satisfied member referrals.

• Carefully calculate the lifetime value and the marginal net worth of your members. These numbers will help you market your club more effectively as well as serve your members more appropriately. You'll know exactly what you can and must spend to get, satisfy, and keep your members for life.

• Service is governed by the rule of 10s. If it costs you $1,000 to get a new member, it takes only 10 seconds to lose one and up to 10 years to overcome the direct and indirect losses resulting from that member leaving.

The Cost of Poor Service

Have you ever sat down to figure out what poor customer service is costing you? Most companies have no idea how much money they're losing or leaving on the table because of poor service. Although they have heard, and I've already told you, that it costs five to six times more to acquire a new customer than it does to conduct business with a current or former customer, these businesses (Is your club one of them?) have no idea about the flip side of that equation: the cost of poor service.

The formula in figure 1.2 developed by the U.S. Office of Consumer Affairs will help you calculate the cost of providing poor service in your club business. To complete the formula, you need to know three figures: your annual revenues, the number of members you have, and the cost of acquiring and keeping those members (including marketing, advertising, the cost of sales, promotions, discounts, and so on). When you complete the formula, feel free to use either dollar amounts or percentages. Either way, you'll get an eye-opening picture of how expensive poor customer service is to your club business.

Lifetime Value of a Member

Now you are aware of how much money it costs your club to get a member and how much it costs your club to lose a member. If you haven't completed

THE COST OF POOR SERVICE

Lost Customer Revenue

A. Annual revenue $\qquad$ \$_____

B. Total number of members _____

C. Percentage of dissatisfied members $\times .25$

D. Number of dissatisfied members = _____

E. Percentage of dissatisfied members who are
likely to switch $\times .70$

F. Number of dissatisfied members who will switch =_____

G. Average revenue per member (A ÷ B) \$_____

H. Revenue lost through poor service (F × G) \$_____

Lost Opportunity Revenue

I. Number of other people dissatisfied customers tell (F × 10) _____

J. Number of potential customers who buy elsewhere because
of negative word of mouth (assume 1 in 50 tell, or 1 × .02) _____

K. Potential lost revenue (J × G) \$_____

Member Replacement Costs

L. Member acquisition costs (___ percent × A; you can use
66 percent or any number you like here.) \$_____

M. Average cost per customer (L ÷ B) \$_____

N. Replacement cost for lost customers (M × 5) \$_____

Total Costs

O. Total annual costs (H + K + N) \$_____

P. Total cost over member's lifetime of doing business
for 10 years (O × 10) \$_____

FIGURE 1.2 *The cost of poor service*
From Members for Life by Richard Gerson, 1999, Champaign, IL: Human Kinetics, copyright 1999 by
Richard Gerson.

The Cost of Poor Service form, you should do so now before proceeding with the material on lifetime value (LTV). When you know what a member is worth to your club compared to what you will lose in revenues if you keep losing customers because of poor treatment, you'll develop a new appreciation for providing great member service.

In order to know what a member's lifetime value is to your club, you must know the acquisition costs associated with that member. Because it costs approximately five or six times as much to acquire a new member as it does to continue selling to and serving a current or former member, one quick way to look at acquisition costs is to simply multiply the potential lost revenue per member that you calculated (line G) by 5. Of course, this result may not be 100 percent accurate, but it does give you an idea of how much money you may be spending to get a new member into your club and how much you're losing when they walk out the door to a competitor.

Another way to figure out member acquisition costs is to carefully track all your expenditures for marketing, advertising, selling, and promotion and divide that figure by the number of new members each activity generates. This calculation gives you a more accurate picture of your true acquisition costs. It also enables you to calculate the lifetime value of your member as well as that member's marginal net worth. Marginal net worth is a calculation that tells you how much money to spend to acquire a member based on the profit you'll make from their repeat purchases over their lifetime with you.

I will explain these concepts in more detail because they are powerful member service and marketing tools. In fact, your understanding of the lifetime value and marginal net worth concepts can help you grow your club faster than your competitors can. I know several companies that have experienced exponential growth from their understanding and use of these concepts.

Lifetime Value and Marginal Net Worth

Companies in all industries allocate a certain dollar amount or a fixed percentage of revenues to marketing and advertising. They do this because "it's always been done this way." This is definitely a mistake, even though most of your competitors are doing it too. In fact, many *Fortune* 500 companies create their marketing budgets this way, even though it's one of the least effective ways to determine how much money should be spent on customer (member) acquisition. This section explains how to use a more effective method of figuring out how much to spend on getting new customers and leave your competitors wondering what happened as you outmarket and outservice them and grow your club.

Let's say that you track all your marketing expenditures and have correctly determined that it costs you $100 to acquire one new member. This amount may be a lot or a little for your club. It may also be industry standard. It doesn't matter if it's realistic. It's just used here as an example and for ease of calculation. You learn that each member you acquire spends $500 with you on his or her first purchase of a membership. That gives you a gross profit of $400, which is the $500 in revenue minus the cost to acquire that member. For this example, let's say your overhead is 20 percent of your gross revenue; that's another $100. That leaves your net profit as $300 per member for the first year's membership, and that doesn't even include any initiation fees or add-on programs.

Your data show that each member makes three additional purchases from you a year, among pro shop, specialty programs, personal training, and other items, and these purchases total $1,500. So each member spends about $2,000 a year in your club. Again, if you use 20 percent as a rough figure for overhead and cost of goods sold, you still make $1,600 a year from each member.

Plus, your average satisfied member stays with you for five years. If we use five years as the lifetime of the member, their overall lifetime value to you is $10,000 in gross revenue ($500 × 3 purchases a year × 5 years). In years 2 through 5, you're making an additional $100 profit on each membership renewal purchase because there are no new acquisition costs. This means that although your overall lifetime value of a member is $10,000, your marginal net worth of that member is $8,400 (net profit from the $10,000 plus the membership renewals). Now that you understand this concept, you realize that you're already making more money than you originally thought from each member.

You can now decide how much more you're willing to spend to acquire a new member. Before you were spending only $100 to get a new member, but now you can easily spend $300 (your net profit from the first sale which is that member's initial marginal net worth) or even $500 (your gross revenue from the first sale) to get that member. The reason you can do this is because you know that this one member will be worth $10,000 gross and $8,400 in pure profit to you over five years.

I realize that this example does not account for member service costs and some operating costs. The example is provided in order to give you an idea of how you can increase your marketing and member service expenditures to get more new members while satisfying and keeping current members. Even though the numbers used in the example may not match your club's situation, they do portray the concepts of LTV and marginal net worth appropriately. There is one caveat to this whole concept, though. You must provide superior member service to all members to ensure that they keep coming back to you for those five years or more. If the service does not meet and exceed their expectations, you can be sure that they'll take their business elsewhere.

So now you have a little-known secret in your marketing and member service arsenal to retain members for life and grow your club. I can assure you that maybe 1 in 100 or even 1,000 club owners has any idea what these concepts are and how they work. You are now that one, so think about how quickly and successfully you can use these concepts to help you grow your club. Just remember to provide great member service to retain members for life.

Using the concepts of lifetime value and marginal net worth forces you to combine marketing with great member service to get and keep members for life. You get another benefit as well. Customers who stay with you a long time tend to refer more people to you, so your member acquisition costs decrease even more. You then have additional monies to either go out and acquire new members in the future, to provide even greater service to your current members, or to keep as pure profit.

Reasons for Poor Service

Think of yourself as a customer for a moment. That should be easy to do because we are all customers of someone or some business. Do you remember the great service you received from a business or the poor service? Because customer service is my area of expertise, I try to look for the great service encounters. Yet I am also like most people. We can relate more service horror stories than positive experiences, and that's probably because the negative service experiences have a greater impact on us. Because that's the case for me, you, and most people, it's probably also true for your members.

What are some of the reasons you would give for not doing business with a company? Why don't you go to a particular restaurant or clothing store anymore? Why don't you fly a specific airline any more? Do your members have similar reasons for not coming back to you? Have you ever wondered why you used to see someone regularly in the club, but now you don't? You need to seriously consider the reasons you may lose a member.

The following list is another compilation of research from various sources, as well as my own research with clients both in and out of the fitness industry, as to why people receive poor service and stop doing business with a company. The most unbelievable thing to me is that here is a customer trying to give someone money for a product or service, and that business owner (or his or her employee) is doing everything possible to turn off that customer. It just doesn't make any sense, especially when customers are the lifeblood of any business. After all, the only reason you're in business is to get,

Unhappy members vote with their feet.

satisfy, and keep a customer. If you take care of your members, your club business will grow and prosper.

Look at this list of 10 reasons for poor service. Then look at them again (a third time wouldn't hurt). Then ask your employees to review the list. Get their feedback. How many have you experienced? How many have they experienced? How many are happening in your club right now? What can you do about it so that you can keep rather than lose members?

10 Reasons for Poor Customer or Member Service

1. The club does not have a member service philosophy or standards of service performance.

2. The club handles complaints poorly or fails to resolve them to the member's satisfaction.

3. Employees receive little or no customer service or technical skills training.

4. Employees are treated poorly by management, and they, in turn, treat members poorly.

5. Employees have uncaring or negative attitudes toward members and/ or each other.

6. Employees are not empowered to provide great customer service or to make decisions that will best serve and satisfy members.

7. The club owners, managers, and employees do not realize that there are differences in what they perceive they are providing in the way of member service and what the member perceives that he or she is receiving.

8. There is a definite difference in what the club thinks members want and what members actually want.

9. The club decides to treat its members in a certain way or as a group, and the members want to be treated in a different way or as individuals.

10. The club believes their membership provides a certain value to the member, but the member perceives it has a different value.

Now that you've read the list, look at it again. Do you see that four of the reasons have to do with how employees are treated and trained by the company and another four have to do with differences in perceptions between members and the club? In a way, the first two reasons relate to the employees also. Furthermore, all the reasons reflect on management or ownership and its philosophy about operating the club.

So the big question is, what are you going to do about it? How will you remedy any or all of these situations if they are occurring in your club today? What will you do to establish new customer service systems within your club or redesign the current systems and processes you already have? I'm sure you are grateful when a member joins your club and not a competitor's club. After all, it is very easy to switch clubs and transfer memberships in one way, shape, or form. So you have to do everything possible to keep the members happy and not push them out the door to your competitors. You must make customer service work for your members. The way to do that is to establish proactive and member-oriented customer service systems within your club.

Making Customer Service Work for Your Members

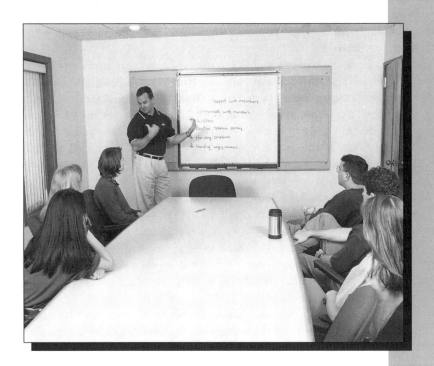

everal years ago, I walked into a health club in Florida. I was planning on joining on the family plan. I stopped at the front desk and waited while the receptionist talked on the phone to someone. And I waited. Then I waited some more. After what seemed like an eternity (but was realistically only about five minutes), I turned around and walked out. Not only did this club lose a member and a family for that initial sale, it lost all the potential money I would have spent in its pro shop, restaurant, juice bar, and on renewals. I wasn't even acknowledged by the receptionist, let alone spoken to. Can you imagine that happening? As I travel to clubs around the country, I see this scene repeated every day.

Think of some companies outside the fitness industry that have advertised superior customer service and have not delivered. Write down the company or the industry on a piece of paper. Here's part of my industry list where companies have talked the talk but forgot to walk the walk of customer service and retention: car dealerships, gas stations, plumbers, electricians, cable TV, restaurants, clothing stores, airlines, music stores, and more. Now, I'm not saying that every business in every industry I've mentioned, or that's on your list, does not deliver on customer service promises. All I'm saying is that certain companies don't deliver. Whose names are on your list? Do you know of any clubs that promise great customer service for their members but don't deliver? Are you one of them?

There is a way that every club can provide great customer service to each of its members all the time. It requires two important things. The first is a corporate culture focused on serving the member to create long-term, loyal members. Everything your club does should be geared to the goal of member retention. Creating this culture involves a concept or process that I call member relationship management (MRM). MRM includes sales, marketing, customer service, retention programs, billing and collections, member communications such as newsletters, and just about anything else that places you or your staff members in contact with members. The MRM process will be explained in greater detail in chapter 10.

The second thing you must do is develop and deliver ongoing training programs in a specific set of skills. When your staff members acquire these skills, they will be able to properly serve and satisfy your members. It is then up to you to empower and enable your staff to go out and serve and satisfy the members.

This training must be more than smile training. It was only a few short years ago that health clubs and companies in other industries began training their employees to provide superior customer service by smiling. That's it. If you smiled at members and nodded in agreement, they would perceive you as someone who was providing superior service, so the theory went. Because club owners were not as educated in customer service as they are now, many of them thought smile training was sufficient. Hopefully, you were not one of those owners then, and you certainly are not one of them now.

It didn't take long for clubs to realize that having employees smile was not enough for members to believe they were receiving great customer service. Other skills were needed, such as the ability to build rapport with members, communicate with them, listen to them, exhibit telephone courtesy, properly manage complaints, and handle angry members. Yet these individual skills would only have a minimal effect on member retention and satisfaction if the club was not doing everything possible to make customer service work. The club management must create the environment and atmosphere in which service-oriented employees can thrive.

Setting Up Customer Service Systems in Your Club

Has this ever happened to you? You've purchased something, and you now have a problem with it. You go back to the store to either return it or get it fixed. You tell your story to the person behind the counter, and he tells you there's nothing he can do about it. You have to talk with the owner or manager or the customer service department, and none of them are available.

Or you call up a company and relate your situation to someone on the phone who, after patiently listening, tells you she can't help you. So she transfers you to someone who can help, you think. You tell your story again only to find out that that person can't help you either. Now, you're starting to get frustrated. You get transferred a third time and get a voice mail message. Now you're really steamed. You vow never to do business with that company again.

In today's business climate, with well-educated and sophisticated customers and more and more competition, it's hard to believe that any business would not have readily accessible customer service systems and people in place. However, I continue to find many businesses, both in and out of the club industry, who make it hard for the customer and easy for themselves. Is your club one of these businesses? Are your customer service systems and processes, policies and procedures, and rules and regulations developed for your benefit or the benefit of your member/customer?

Customer service systems must include staff training.

Many clubs throughout the world are trying to improve their customer service. If you asked club owners, they'd tell you that they are always doing everything possible to serve and satisfy their customers. Yet when you try to get some service, it's either very poor or nonexistent. You don't have to believe me. Have you ever asked your members what they think of your service? I have.

Some are happy, some are not. Others just tolerate whatever level of service you provide. Is that the perception of your club that you want your members to have? One of tolerance? I know I wouldn't want that for my club. I'd want the members to be thrilled to be there, to be strong advocates of my club, and to tell the world about how great my club is. I assume you want that for your club also.

So what are you supposed to do? The answer is very simple. You need to establish customer service systems and processes in your club that welcome members, that make it easy for them to do business with you, and that help them get their problems resolved and questions answered as quickly as possible and to their satisfaction.

Establishing customer service systems takes a great deal of work. Clubs have to invest time and money in the process, which must include staff training, but the process does not have to be that difficult or that expensive. You can establish customer service protocols very easily, as long as you're willing to support the initiative and get your employees behind the movement so it will succeed. Management and ownership support are critical to making customer service work in a club setting, or in any business setting. Just as important is the employee support of the customer service initiative. If the employees are not willing to provide the great service, you and your members will definitely suffer.

I've broken down the development of a customer service system in a company to a simple seven-step process. Follow these seven steps, and you will develop a successful customer service system for your members. Keep in mind that these steps do not have to be followed in any specific order, although the order I'm presenting them in will get you the best and quickest results. You should follow these steps regardless of whether you're a single location club or you have multiple facilities, whether you are a single purpose or multipurpose facility, and whether you are for profit or not for profit.

Seven Steps to an Effective Club Customer Service System

1. **Have total management commitment.** The club owner, the management staff, and the entire support staff must be committed to making customer service work for the members. Management cannot just give lip service to customer service. They must walk the walk and support the staff in their efforts to provide superior customer service that builds member loyalty. Furthermore, managers and owners must be so committed to the customer service initiative that they "imbue" it into the corporate culture.

If you're like most club owners, you know that you'll never get really rich in the club business, so you must be doing it for other reasons. One major reason is to positively impact the lives of your members through service. Your club mission, vision, values, and purpose statements must reflect this focus on the member. Your marketing strategies and tactics, along with your daily operating procedures, must be aligned to serve and satisfy the customers. Your entire management staff must also fully support your other staff members in their efforts to take care of the club members.

2. **Know your members.** Learn everything you can about your members. Conduct surveys, interviews, and focus groups. Get to know their families, friends, and business associates. Find out what your members like and dislike, learn their primary reasons for joining your club, uncover any reasons that may cause them to leave, and then educate everyone on staff with this information about your members.

The best thing to do is to place all this information in your member database and make it readily accessible to your entire staff. In my experiences as a consultant in the club industry, I have found many facilities that are not using their computerized "front desk" programs to the fullest possible extent. If you collect the right information, input it properly, and update it as needed, then you have a warehouse full of important information on each member.

You need to study that information to learn as much as you can about everyone who joins your club. Can you imagine the positive boost in a member's self-esteem when you go up to her and ask about her child's birthday, or how his new cross-training program affected his job performance, or how much body fat she's lost after being on a specially designed program? When you have all this information available in your database, you look like a genius who cares about his or her members.

3. **Develop standards of performance for customer service.** If you don't measure it, you'll never improve it. When you first opened your club, you probably developed job descriptions and standards of performance related to those job descriptions. If you're like most businesses, those standards were for observable task behaviors related to performing the job rather than serving the customer. To make customer service work in your club, you must develop service standards of performance, identify how they can be measured, and then measure them precisely. Each job should have its own service standards. The club itself should also have a series of service standards that everyone must meet or exceed.

The standards are important to service success because they give the staff something to shoot for. After all, how many basketball games have you played where you didn't keep score? How interesting would fitness competitions be if there were no winners, just performers? The answers are not many and not very. You need to keep some type of score to let people know how they are doing. Keeping score (measuring performance results) tends to motivate people to greater achievements. Wouldn't you like your staff to be known as the best service providers in the entire industry?

The purpose of these standards and the measurement system you use to evaluate them is to improve your service delivery to members, not to find out what your staff is doing wrong. You must communicate this fact to them. You are not looking over their shoulders for mistakes. You are looking for ways to improve everyone's service to the members. If a staff member is performing poorly, then remedial steps must be taken. You cannot let this slip by. You establish service standards of performance that must be met so you will have long-term member retention, so you must take the appropriate steps to improve everyone's performance. A poor performance indicates a training need as well as an opportunity to improve efforts that lead to member retention.

4. **Hire, train, and compensate good, service-oriented staff.** You can't train niceness, but you can hire nice people. Sure, it's great to get people with experience for whatever position you hire them, but you can always train for positional skills. You can never train for niceness. That's why you must select service-oriented people who possess the technical skills you need.

No matter what your employees' backgrounds are or how nice they are, you train them to provide the highest level of quality service possible. This training includes service skills training, corporate mission and culture training, and even member relationship management process training. After all, everyone on your staff should know exactly how his or her job contributes to the success of the club, which is based on successfully serving and retaining members.

Once you have a quality staff member, compensate that person appropriately. Although money may not be the prime motivator for some people, and you should ask staff members individually how important money is to them, it is still a strong motivator. Proper compensation for a job well done leads to more satisfied and longer term employees, which, in turn, leads to better service for your members. The relationship is very simple: The greater your employee retention, the greater your member retention tends to be. That's because members establish relationships and alliances with employees. Sometimes, their loyalty is more to your employees than to the club. Remember the story in chapter 1 about the morning receptionist who knew everyone's name? You can bet those members were more loyal to her than to the club or anyone else.

Talk to your members. If your club experiences repeated turnover in any of your departments, especially the front desk, ask your members how they feel about that. They will tell you that they don't enjoy seeing new faces every time they come in to work out. They don't care what your problems are in hiring or retaining competent personnel—they just want the comfort of knowing that they will see the same faces each time they come in.

Take this question to another level. How do your members feel if their personal trainer(s) keeps leaving your club? Remember that a psychological and an emotional attachment develops between your members and your staff. To retain your members, you must do everything possible to keep your staff intact.

5. **Reward service accomplishments.** Several years ago, a club general manager came to me and asked how she could motivate her employees without paying them additional compensation. I suggested gold stars—that's right, the kind of gold stars you used to get in kindergarten and first grade when you did something well. Of course, she thought I was crazy. After all, why would adults be motivated to perform if all they were going to receive in return was a gold star?

I asked her to try it for two weeks and then get back to me with her results. After two weeks, she came by to see me and presented me with my own gold star. She said that the program worked so well, she couldn't believe it. The employees were comparing how many gold stars they earned, and a few friendly competitions began.

What does this example tell us? It tells us that everyone appreciates being appreciated for what they do. We all have a need for reward and recognition. As an owner, manager, or colleague, it is up to you to fulfill that need for other employees. When someone does a good job, acknowledge that performance. You can give them a gold star; you can put a mark on a wall chart; or you can verbally praise them. Whatever you do, let them know that you appreciate their efforts and you're willing to make a big deal about how well they're doing.

When you reinforce a behavior in a positive manner, that behavior gets repeated. Remember that reward and recognition programs don't have to be monetary. The club can offer the employee travel incentives, shopping certificates, paid days off from work, massages and facials, telephone calling cards, baby-sitting services, housecleaning service, and many more things to serve as a reward.

Establish your reward and recognition programs and make your staff feel good about providing great service to members. Also, make as big a public display of these recognition and reward efforts as you can. It will help build the self-esteem of your employees and make them want to provide even better service to the members.

You should also reward and recognize your members for their good behaviors. When they wipe off the equipment; when they refer new members into the club; or when they help out another member, recognize their efforts, and you'll see how quickly they repeat those same positive behaviors. You may even want to mention these member actions in your club newsletter.

In one club I worked with several years ago, we created a Good Member chart. To get your name on the chart, you had to be seen by a staff member wiping down the equipment after you used it, helping other members with their workouts, or doing other things that showed you were a good citizen. Every week, we put the names of members on a chart that was visible in the workout area. Many members laughed at the idea at first. But after a while, they started asking how they could get their names on the chart. We gave them the criteria, and they started doing everything possible to get on and stay on the Good Member chart. Reward your employees and members; the benefits are unlimited.

6. **Communicate with your members.** To retain members, you must stay in constant communication with them. Be proactive and send them newsletters, post flyers, have a bulletin board, talk with them regularly, and hold member councils and member advisory meetings. Send them special mailings or special offers on club programs and services. Call them up to thank them for using your club on a regular basis. Call them up and ask them where they've been if they haven't been into the club for a while. Or just call them up to say hello.

These "hello, how are you" calls, as I call them, are very powerful in cementing your relationships with your members. Members appreciate the time you're taking to contact them, especially because you're not trying to sell them anything. That's another important point—if the only time you communicate with members is when you want to sell them another program, product, or service, then they will start to resent you and your club. They'll think all you want to do is put your hand in their pockets and come away with more money.

Talk to your members.

You need to show them you care about them. Hold parties and social events for them. Host a dinner. Give a member a birthday party or a graduation party, or have members hold one of their civic club meetings at your facility. Tell them, write them, and show them all these things. Make sure you communicate with them in every way possible. If your members have an e-mail address, get it from them and send them e-mails on club happenings. Create an e-zine or an e-letter for them on a monthly basis. Make your communications proactive and interesting.

Do whatever you must to stay close to your members and to keep them feeling important. Communicate that you care more often than you communicate club information. This communication will go a long way to retaining them psychologically and physically. Many times, the psychological relationship you establish with a member is more important than the financial one when it comes to member retention.

7. **Continuously improve service.** Never rest on your laurels. When you think you have this customer service thing down pat, another club goes you one better. Whatever you do today, find a way to improve it tomorrow. Benchmark your current performance against the performance of other facilities.

Go outside the industry and find out what a Four Seasons Hotel or Ritz-Carlton does to serve their guests. Check out different restaurants to see how they serve and treat customers. Identify the best in different service industries and see how you can adapt your processes and systems to achieve that status.

Help your staff improve also. Measure and evaluate each person's performance and then help him or her improve his or her abilities. Provide staff members with additional training in job-related skills, technical skills, people skills, fitness information, and career planning. Help them become more than they are. Work on their self-esteem. Remember that for both of you, good enough is never truly good enough. Always ask what you and they can and must do to get better.

Don't end up like a club I was called in to help that did a customer service survey of their members. The results of the survey showed that the club was providing the type of service and offering the programs that the members wanted. Unfortunately, the survey really didn't measure the level of service, so the level of service never improved. As a result, members started leaving. Obviously, things were not as fine as the survey seemed to indicate.

The way I helped the club was to interview the members in focus groups and find out what they wanted and expected in the way of customer service. I then took the club through the previous six steps to create that type of service atmosphere and trained the staff in customer service skills, such as interpersonal communication, listening, and telephone courtesy. All these skills will be covered in more detail in subsequent chapters.

SEVEN STEPS TO AN EFFECTIVE CLUB CUSTOMER SERVICE SYSTEM

1. Have total management commitment.

2. Know your members.

3. Develop standards of performance for customer service.

4. Hire, train, and compensate good, service-oriented staff.

5. Reward service accomplishments.

6. Communicate with your members.

7. Continuously improve service.

Training Makes Customer Service Work for Your Members

I've mentioned training twice in the last few paragraphs. It's been my experience that clubs do not provide enough customer service training for their employees. Most of the training focuses on membership sales, ancillary programs that generate revenues, and personal training. Of course, everyone should be trained in these important areas. After all, if you don't sell a membership or a program, you won't have a club.

Yet it's also important to train your staff in customer service skills and customer relationship management techniques. Be aware that the service and the management of the member relationship is what keeps members coming back. If your staff is not skilled in these approaches, your members will go elsewhere to get the kind of treatment they want and expect.

Club owners are always concerned about whether they can afford this type of training. Yes, training is an up-front expense, but it is also an eventual revenue generator. So regardless of what training programs may cost you up front, can you really afford not to train your staff?

Service Strategy Alignment

One of the most important areas to train your staff in is the club's service philosophy and strategy, along with your mission, vision, values, purpose, and culture. All these things may seem like a lot to teach employees, but unless they know and understand what you mean by each of these things, they'll never truly be able to provide the levels of service you expect of them.

Take a look at your club's mission statement. If it reads something like "To be the premier provider of health and fitness services . . . " or "To positively impact people's lifestyles and enhance their well-being . . .," get rid of it! You need a mission statement that expands your purpose and reason for being. To create this mission statement, first read the mission statements of other clubs and other companies, and then ask people about their own personal mission statements. Then take the best of everything and modify it to fit your club setting.

1. Read the mission statements of other clubs and other companies outside the fitness industry.

2. Ask people about their own personal mission statements.

3. Ask your members why they joined your club.

4. Ask your members what they expect from you as a service provider.

5. Write your mission statement to describe your purpose for being in business and how you plan to serve your customers.

6. Take the best of everything you've read and learned, modify it to fit your club setting, and update your original mission statement.

7. Test it out on your employees and members to see if they fully understand what you mean that you plan to do.

Our mission statement at Gerson Goodson Performance Management is to help clients improve the performances of their employees, maximize productivity, and turn ordinary performers into extraordinary performers.

Make sure your mission statement is different from your vision statement. Your vision statement is where or what you want your club to be in 5 years (or 10). The mission statement will help you achieve your vision. Similarly, your purpose is what gets you up in the morning. What are you passionate about with respect to your club? What gets you going and keeps you going? When you define your purpose with a passion, then you'll know you're on the right road to success.

The last thing you must create in your service strategy is your value set. What are the values you hold dear, and how do you communicate them to your staff? How do you let the members know about your values? How do you align your values with your behaviors?

When you have all these things in place, then you can align your mission, vision, values, and purpose to create your corporate culture. This culture will reflect how well your service strategy is aligned. Without this alignment, meaning that all employees are on the same page and moving in the same direction, your club will barely get along.

I've had the pleasure of working with several hospitals and their wellness centers these past years. Hospitals are extremely focused on establishing their mission, vision, and values and then aligning them to form a service strategy. My work involved helping the wellness centers translate the hospital strategy into the wellness center strategy. In every case, all behaviors and efforts were focused on the patient/member/customer. When we trained the staff on the mission, vision, and values of the wellness center, they were easily able to manage their customer relationships. Satisfaction levels improved, as did the working environment. Obviously there are both direct and indirect benefits from aligning your service strategy.

Here's a personal example from my company. With respect to our work in performance management, and specifically customer relationship management, which combines the disciplines of sales, marketing, customer service, information technology, and training, we have positioned ourselves as The Customer Relationship Management Company. Our vision is to be the premier provider of CRM consulting services to companies both in and out of the fitness industry within the next five years. Our mission is to build businesses by helping them build better long-term relationships with their customers.

The values we hold dear include love, family, health, honesty, integrity, open communication, credit where credit is due, fun, creativity, and support of people. While this list is not in priority order, the first several are in order. This is how our company is run, how our service strategies are aligned, and how we treat our customers, competitors, and employees.

Accessibility

To make customer service work in your facility, you must consider this question: "How accessible are the customer service systems within my club?" To answer this big question, you first need to ask a more specific question: "How easy is it for members to complain, change their membership status, get information, make a purchase, or cancel their membership?" Accessibility refers to how easy it is for members to ask for service, receive service, and then feel they are satisfied with the service they receive.

Say a member calls up the billing department of a club and asks for information regarding his or her account status. The person answering the phone tells the member that he is not authorized to give out that information. He then asks the member to call back. Suppose a member calls up a club and reaches the front desk receptionist. The member is calling to either renew or upgrade a membership. The receptionist tells the member that no salesperson is available and asks the member to call back. What if a member wants to talk to a personal trainer about the program and its costs, and all your personal trainers are either busy or not in the club? The member has to wait for another time or come back at a later date.

I could go on and on, but I'm sure you get the picture. These three examples are negative, yet they accurately describe what goes on in clubs today regarding accessibility to customer service systems. Members are constantly being put off, put on hold on the phone, or told to take their complaints to the manager. Complaint management and accessibility is covered in its own chapter (chapter 6) because handling complaints is so important to your success. For now, realize that one of the most important keys to customer service success is being accessible to your members.

Many clubs and companies in other industries have a set of policies and procedures manuals. They give their employees a copy of these manuals, ask them to study them and learn them, and even test them on the contents. Then, they tell the employees to perform their jobs in accordance with the policies and procedures set forth in the manuals.

And that, my friends, is the major problem. The policies and procedures are usually written for the benefit of the company and its employees. In reality, they should be written to make everything easier for the customer/member. The one thing members never want to hear is that you can't do something for them because it's against company policy.

Establish your guidelines, policies, and procedures and follow them, to a point. Remember that they are guidelines, not rules set in concrete. Teach them to your employees, but make sure your employees know that they can make independent decisions to serve and satisfy the customer. Your policies and procedures must be adaptable and flexible so your employees can apply them to individual situations. Each member comes to you with his or her own set of needs and problems. No one can predict all the things that can occur during the daily operation of a club. That means that not everything can be covered in your policies and procedures manuals. So when a new or unique situation comes up, what does your employee do?

Let members know you care.

If you run a rigid club that must adhere to its policies and procedures, your employees will be forced to tell the member they cannot help him or her. If you run a service-oriented club, then your employees will use the policies and procedures as guides to help them make the appropriate decisions to serve the member. You can do everything mentioned in this chapter to make customer service work for your members. But the first time an employee denies a member's request for something because it's not in your rule book, everything else you've done related to providing great customer service is negated. You'll have to start all over again to make customer service work in your club for your members.

Once you establish customer service systems in your club, there are two other things you should do. The first is to post the results of everyone's service efforts. Make a chart or charts of performance and post them where the employees can see them daily. Some clubs even put them out on the workout floor, so the members can see how well everyone is doing. The chart's location is up to you. The important thing is that the chart publicly identifies measurements of performance and areas for improvements.

The second thing is to make all your customer service systems accessible, easy to use, and member-friendly. The last thing you want is for members to have problems or need some information and have no way of getting what they need taken care of. You must make the club work for the members. They are your only reason for being in business. Your customer service systems must make the members' lives easier, not yours. This approach may be a hard pill to swallow, but it will increase your member retention and profits. And those are the reasons you're in business: to get, satisfy, and keep members for life so that your club business remains profitable.

In a nutshell, here are seven things you must do to make customer service work to retain members in your club:

1. Develop a corporate service philosophy and service strategy.
2. Align the service strategy with your mission, vision, values, and purpose.
3. Train your staff to deliver exceptional customer service to members.
4. Make your policies and procedures easy for the members instead the staff.
5. Make your service systems easily accessible to members.
6. Develop a complaint management and service recovery system that focuses on satisfying members and then exceeding their expectations for the situation (more on this topic later in the book).
7. Do what works all over again and try to make it better.

CHAPTER 3

What Members Really Need, Want, and Expect

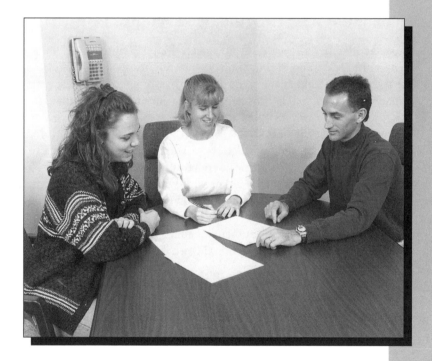

Has this ever happened to you? You're operating your club, and things seem to be fine. The members aren't complaining, the staff seems happy, and cash is flowing. Life seems great. You haven't heard anything negative from the members, so you figure that you're giving them what they need and want.

Boy, are you under a grave misconception! Just because you haven't heard a complaint from your members does not mean that they are completely happy with the service you're providing. One of the major gaps that occurs in customer service is that the service provider, in this case, you as the club owner, believes that the business is providing one level of service, but the customer or member perceives that he or she is receiving a lower level of service. Just because no one complains or voices his opinion doesn't make what you're doing right.

In fact, only 4 percent of your members will ever complain at any given time. Most of them will suffer silently and eventually walk away. That's one of the reasons that the attrition rate in the club industry is at 40 percent or more. It's up to you and all your employees to close this service gap. You must provide superior member service as your members perceive it.

Superior Member Service: A Definition

Superior member service does not mean doing things right. Doing things right is efficiency. Superior member service requires you to be effective; to do the right things right at the right time. If this sounds like it's just a matter of semantics, think again. It's not semantics in your members' minds. They want you to do what's right for them and by them as they define it.

Remember that the definitions of quality service and member satisfaction are the same: Quality and satisfaction are whatever the member says they are. Your own definition of superior service may be very admirable. But it is worthless unless it completely aligns with your members' definitions. Their definitions of quality customer service will be based on their needs, wants, and expectations.

You must know exactly what members need from you, what they want as a result of doing business with you, and what they expect throughout their membership term and your ongoing relationship with them. Every member needs, wants, and expects different things, which makes your task all the more difficult. What if you have 1,000 members? Or 5,000

Provide superior member service as members perceive it.

members? Or even 10,000 members? How will you ever find out exactly what each member needs from you? There is only one way to get the information you need: You must ask them.

That's right. You must ask each and every member exactly what they expect in the way of service, performance results (weight loss, strength, or cardiovascular gains, for example), and treatment by your staff. A good idea is to ask them before they join, again when they join, and periodically during their membership. Make sure that every time one of your staff members gathers this information, it is included in your database so your entire workforce can access it at any time.

Because many clubs have a great many members, and this task is quite large, the clubs forego it for the sake of convenience. That is one of the biggest mistakes they can make. You can't give members what they need, want, and expect if you're taking the easy way out by doing what's convenient for you and your staff. You must accept the responsibility to become informed.

When you don't get the information firsthand, you become like so many other clubs that think they know exactly what their members want. They make assumptions based on industry data, past experiences, or their own preferences. They decide that this misinformation is appropriate and correct, so they go out and give the members their interpretation of great service. Unfortunately, most of the time, clubs guess wrong. Now, they are either in trouble or out of business altogether. Never be naive enough or arrogant enough to presume you can read the minds of your members.

You don't have to assume anything in the fitness industry or club business. All you have to do is ask your members what they need, want, and expect from you, and they'll be happy to tell you. They may tell you more than you want to hear, but that is fine. The more information you have from them and about them, the more you are able to serve them properly.

If you don't have any members yet because you are just starting out, ask the members of your future competitors what they want in the way of great member/customer service. They'll be only too happy to tell you. You'll learn what's right and wrong with your competitors' clubs. You'll learn what you need to do to please members. You'll also learn what marketing and sales messages you must send to get these people to become members of your club. This information becomes a competitive advantage that you can use.

For example, when members of a competitor's club tell you they want certain things they're not getting, you've just uncovered some unmet needs on the part of your competitor. When you show you can serve, meet, and satisfy those needs for those members, you'll win the members over to your club. You may even want to offer the members of your competitors a trial membership at your club. Emphasize the benefits of the specific services you offer that satisfy their unmet needs. Play them up big and have your staff play them up big. Do whatever it takes to show those people that they belong at your club where they'll get the level of service they expect and deserve.

Basic Member (and Human) Needs

All members have the 10 needs revealed in the following list in one capacity or another. This list is neither complete nor perfect for your particular club. You should modify it, add and delete items, and adapt it to make it work for your club. Remember that this list is just a starting point and it is based on my extensive experience and research in the customer service and marketing arenas of over 100 different industries, including fitness and health clubs. Members (and customers) need the following from you:

Help

Respect and recognition

Comfort, compassion, and support

To be listened to with empathy

Service that leads to satisfaction

Trust and trustworthiness

A friendly, smiling face

Understanding

To be made to feel important

A quality product or service at a fair price

These are some of the things members need from you. There are definitely other things they want in addition to these. Don't confuse the two items. Needs are "got to have" things, and wants are "nice to have" things. For example, if you have holes in your workout clothes, you need some new clothes. You may want an expensive outfit, but that's not what you need. You need a simple set of workout clothes. Similarly, if your equipment is outdated, you need to replace it. You may want to replace it with the latest and greatest technological marvels, but that's not what you need. You need equipment that gets the job done for your members.

These examples make the difference very clear. Needs are more tangible; wants are more psychological. The difference is more than semantic; it is very real. As far as your members are concerned, just ask them what they need and want from you. They'll tell you, and if they confuse needs and wants, it's your job to ask for clarification.

Meeting and Exceeding Member Expectations

The other area you must be clear on relates to member expectations of you. Members possess certain criteria for successful performance, and they define these criteria by establishing expectations. Expectations refer to how well you meet their objectives and standards for success or excellent service performance.

Expectations have nothing to do with you or what you're doing from your perspective. They are solely the perception of the member. Suppose your club policy is to return all member phone calls within 24 hours. You post this policy in the member handbook, and you've told the members about this policy when they joined. In your mind, you've done a good job of trying to manage member expectations. But a member calls in with some issue that is very important to her and expects a call back within two hours. She even leaves this message on your voice mail or with a staff member. Due to other commitments, you call her the next day. You have clearly responded within your stated club policy. But you've also clearly not met her expectations.

No amount of explaining about your policies or even apologizing is going to change that member's perception that her expectation was not met. She may forgive you (this time), but that doesn't mean she will do so a second time. Ask yourself how that member feels about your behavior and the fact that you didn't "keep your promise." Yes, I know you didn't promise the member directly that you'd call back within two hours. But, in her mind, that promise was made because she left you that message, and her need was important. So she expected you to meet her requirements, and you didn't do so.

> **Ask your members what they want.**

Think about how you feel when you're waiting for a table in a restaurant or are in line for a movie. You're told it will be only 15 minutes, and you're still waiting 30 minutes later. Your expectations of wait time have not been met, and you're beginning to have a variety of negative thoughts about this restaurant or movie. Even when you're seated, you begin the evening with a negative attitude that affects your entire experience. This is exactly what happens to your members when you fail to meet their expectations of a level of service that they "demand" from you.

To determine your members' expectations of doing business with you, you must ask them directly. You can use personal interviews, focus groups, telephone interviews, written surveys, or other types of questionnaires. The proper development and application of these tools are discussed in detail in my book, *Measuring Customer Satisfaction* (Crisp Publications, 1993). You must do something to get your members to communicate their expectations to you.

Determining How to Satisfy Members

First, you must understand that member satisfaction is now the baseline for success. It used to be that if you met customers' expectations, you could conclude that they would be satisfied. You could also be assured of doing well in business. Now we know that satisfaction is merely the ante to get into the game. Because everyone is providing a high level of customer service, and people change providers quite frequently, you've got to do more to keep your members. You've got to go beyond meeting their expectations to exceeding their expectations.

You've got to find out what's going on in their heads and their hearts. Questioning the members will give you some insight into what they need, want, and expect of you. You must also examine your own business. A self-analysis of your business will help you determine your strengths and deficiencies and will also enable you to improve your service to your members.

Ask yourself these five questions about your members and your club to determine how you think they perceive doing business with you:

1. What result or benefit will members receive from belonging to my club?

2. What is a member's need level for my programs and services?

3. How important is membership in my club to members based on the needs or the wants satisfied by their membership?

4. What are the perceived costs and perceived risks the member has related to belonging to my club?

5. What does the member want me to do to maintain his or her loyalty to my club?

Now go out and ask these same questions of all your members. Put the responses in your database so everyone has access to them. After you, your staff, and your members have answered these questions, you'll have a pretty good idea of how to satisfy your members. You'll know the exact behaviors you and your staff must provide to meet and exceed member expectations. You'll also know how members will judge your performance. Plus, you'll be able to determine your areas for improvement based on the differences among the answers of the three responding groups.

Of course, your best knowledge will come from asking members exactly what they expect of you. By the way, if you've figured out that I'm repeating myself, you're right. It must be said over and over again. The only way to know exactly what you must do to satisfy your members is to ask them directly. Ask this question, face-to-face: "What exactly do you expect from the club in the way of programs, services, and personal treatment?"

It used to be that if you provided good member service, members would seek you out instead of your competitors. In the mid-'80s, I worked with a new club that just opened but did not have the latest or greatest equipment at the time. It was also in the geographic marketing area of two of the major chains. The club management and I focused on training the staff to treat the members as people instead of numbers. We also promoted this fact in the club's marketing and advertising. Membership grew to 90 percent of capacity within 18 months.

Then the large chain clubs in the area started improving their service. Service could no longer be used as a differentiating factor to sell memberships, for my client or anyone else. So we came up with other ways to enhance both the programs the club provided and the member service that went along with them. We called this *value-added service*. At the time, we did little things such as offer free baby-sitting. We developed specialty classes that we didn't charge for, although today many clubs require a fee for these non-dues revenue programs. Some other examples of value-added service you may be familiar with include a free personal training session upon joining, a free massage, or home personal training services.

You may be offering a wide variety of value-added services. You're meeting and exceeding the expectations of your members. The only problem is that your competitors can catch up quickly. Now, as I said before, when a club is capable of meeting a member's expectations of service, that is only the ante into the game. You no longer hold all the chips or high cards. Good, even great member service only lets you stay in the game and levels the playing field between large and small clubs or single-purpose and multipurpose clubs. To be successful and to keep members for life, you've got to provide "greater than great" member and customer service. You've got to consistently exceed members' expectations, so members come away from each workout at your club saying wow! Quite simply, you've got to dazzle and delight your members every chance you get.

How to Dazzle and Delight Members to Get to the Wow Factor

Members are delighted when you do something for them that they never expected. For example, if people have the old-time perception that when they come in to join a club they will be herded into a small closing room (similar to some automobile dealerships), then that is their expectation. But when you take them on a walking tour, or into a restaurant, or into a conference room to discuss their membership plan, they are wowed. They never expected this, and they are more than pleased to receive this "special" treatment.

You've got to start this process of dazzling and delighting your members well before you first interact with them. You need to improve your awareness of certain things related to members and member service, as well as develop an understanding of common member behaviors. Although the following information is somewhat generic, it is applicable to most, if not all, of your members, and it's based on over 20 years experience in this industry.

Let's begin your wow training with developing and increasing your awareness. Superior service providers are aware of many things, sometimes too numerous to mention. The list on page 41 shows 15 things that affect member service that you must always be aware of. When you review them and make them part of your repertoire, you'll have a head start on your competition. The list is applicable for club owners, managers, and employees, as well as members who have to interact with staff and other members.

I've also included blank spaces at the end of the list for you to customize it to your particular club. I strongly recommend you fill in those items and clarify or describe them. You must also share them with your staff. Don't look upon this exercise as a tedious task; it is the basis for many profit-producing internal marketing activities as well as the development of positive, long-term member relationships.

You should increase your awareness and perception in all these areas. Pay attention to as many items on the list as possible. When you do, your members will appreciate the personal interest you take in them. All these factors go into how a member perceives and judges your club with regard to service and renewal. It's up to you to create the right impression. Combine your knowledge of these items with many of the other recommendations in the book, and your members will be shouting Wow! every time they come to work out.

How to Handle Different Types of Members

Now that you have an idea of how to create the wow factor, you've got to understand how members will behave when they do business with you. You will encounter at least the following 10 behavior patterns from members; you probably can identify many more. This list is again compiled to give you the benefit of my 20-plus years of experience in the industry and to get you started thinking about these issues. Ask yourself what you must do to work with and satisfy each type of member. More specifically, after you read each description, ask yourself "How will I handle that type of member?"

The Superior, Know-It-All Member

This person knows your business better than you do and will not hesitate to tell you and anyone else who will listen. Most often, she will tell you what you're doing wrong, even when you do things right. She will also make as many attempts as possible to prove you and your staff wrong. Members of this type are a case of egos out of control with a definite need to prove their superiority.

The Resistant Member

No matter what you try to do for this person, he will resist every effort on your part to satisfy him. He will tell you what he wants from you, and then when you give it to him, he'll tell you it's either wrong or no good. Members of this type do whatever they can to break club rules and not adhere to

FACTORS AFFECTING SERVICE

In order to provide great member service and begin to keep members for life, you need to be aware of the following things in yourself, your colleagues, and your members:

Attitudes

Behaviors

Concerns

Desires, wants, and wishes

Expectations and intentions

Perceptions

Physical state

Mental and emotional state

How the physical state is affecting mental state and vice versa

Influencers, such as family and friends

Personal appearance

Club appearance and environment

Communication

Availability and accessibility of staff

Costs of doing business and providing service

_____

_____

_____

_____

_____

policies and procedures. It's as if they thoroughly enjoy making themselves and others miserable, or at least stressing people out.

The Dependent Member

This member is like a newborn infant that is totally dependent on a parent. This type of member wants you to do everything for her and will not lift a finger to help herself. She wants your staff to guide her through each workout, to reassure her that everything is OK, and to practically beg her to come back. Dependent members also have a need to be needed, and they may ask your staff to prove it at every opportunity.

The Hostile/Antagonistic Member

This member loves to pick a fight or an argument or simply wants to stir up things. It's not that members of this type are having a bad day; they're usually having a bad life, and they take it out on everyone they meet. Be careful, because this member can become verbally and physically abusive with your staff and other members. When you combine this behavior pattern with the Resistant Member pattern, you have someone you must really watch out for. He can destroy your entire club and any harmony you may have built up among the members and staff.

The Depressed Member

Nothing you do satisfies this type of member. You would think that exercise would be the best antidepressant there is. Unfortunately, some people just are unhappy. Their lives are miserable. (Yes, you and I both know that in most of these cases, their misery is a choice.) Yet you have to have pity for anyone who is always sad. If you decide to spend time listening to this member's problems, do not become her therapist. She will take up so much of your time that you won't be available to help anyone else. Plus, becoming her "therapist" will drain your own energies.

The Uncommunicative Member

It's hard to know how to satisfy someone when he doesn't tell you what you need to know. Members of this type don't answer your questions; they don't respond to surveys; and they don't talk to anyone on the staff. They choose to be uncommunicative and may even revel in their silence. In this case, though, their silence is deafening, and it could be deadly to retain them as a member.

The Talkative Member

This member is just the opposite of the uncommunicative member. She never seems to shut up. Although members of this type probably just want someone to listen to them, their constant talking can become annoying. These are the people who are still talking while you're trying to explain their membership categories to them or who talk while the personal trainer is teaching them about equipment. After a while, their constant chatter becomes torture, like a dripping faucet. You must develop a way to quiet them down without insulting them, making them feel disrespected, or shattering their self-esteem.

The Let-Others-Speak-for-Me Member

This person won't say a word to you, but he has other members, friends, and family act as the intermediaries or messengers. He may also have difficulty making decisions. This type of member is a follower, so be careful not to let him be influenced by another member who is negative.

The Chronic Complainer

Everyone knows this member. Although this member is probably a combination of several of the other types, she deserves separate mention. Members of this type buy, complain, and return what they bought. Or they want a refund. Or they want an extension on their membership. Or they just want to chew your head off. Or they want to test you to see how well and quickly you respond to their complaints. Whatever you do for them, they're never going to be happy with you or your club. The only time they're really ever happy is when they're complaining and making someone else's life miserable.

The Perfect Member

This person buys from you and is so satisfied with the purchase, he refers your club to other people. Members of this type become your advocates, apostles, and best unpaid sales force. They are thrilled with what you and your staff are doing for them and truly appreciate the life-affirming changes they are experiencing at your club. If and when they complain, it is to provide you with feedback so you can improve your service to them the next time.

Find your perfect members; ask them what they love about doing business with you, and use this information in your marketing and service materials; and then ask them for referrals. Do whatever you can and must to keep these members happy, satisfied, and loyal. Also, ask them to serve as ombudsmen on behalf of your club to other members. Sometimes, a member can resolve another member's problem better than a staff person can. This creation of a community within the club definitely helps your member retention efforts.

You must be aware of these 10 different types of member behaviors in order to more effectively provide members with what they need, want, and expect from you. Train yourself and your staff how to identify each type and how to handle each type. It's important for everyone to know what to do because you will encounter these people several times each day. Don't run away from them because members are the lifeblood of your business. Regardless of their behavior patterns, find out what their individual expectations are and then determine how to meet and exceed them. Do whatever it takes, within reason, to dazzle and delight them. When they join your club and come for their workout, have them leave every time saying Wow!

Give Members the NEWS

One of your goals as you try to improve member retention in your club is to determine what members need (N), expect (E), and want (W). You also need to ask your members what satisfies (S) them. Ask them to be as specific as possible. When you know what satisfies them, you can do whatever you must to give it to them. When you give your members the NEWS, they'll be sure to stick around.

Let's say that a group of your members is pleased with your club, but they don't seem overly enthused. This is the perfect time to ask them exactly what you must do to satisfy them. They may say that they want more towel stands available throughout the club, or that the front desk area should be brighter, or that your staff should do a better job of learning and remembering everyone's name. It doesn't matter whether you agree with them; you've got to give them what satisfies them. Find out what they need, expect, and want and then dazzle and delight them. That helps satisfy them perceptually. Now you must find out what satisfies them behaviorally and give it to them. These actions will help you start to retain your members for life.

Members as Raters

By now, you should be totally convinced of the importance of serving and satisfying members' needs, wants, and expectations. If not, here's another reason. Whenever you interact with members, they rate you. You may not know exactly what standards or criteria members are using, and they may not even know, but one thing you can be sure of: The member is rating every encounter, meeting, and workout related to their perceived level and quality of service. They also rate you according to their own level of satisfaction with the entire interaction, and then they transfer this perception to their overall evaluation of your club.

You know this is true because of what you do every time you buy something. You review the situation and consider how you were greeted, how the salesperson or clerk or trainer spoke to you, and how that person treated you throughout the entire encounter. Then you form an impression of the company you're doing business with. That impression may be positive or negative, and it will determine how often you decide to do business with the company again. You do it, I do it, and your members do it.

Several years ago, Zeithaml, Parasuraman, and Berry investigated the parameters customers use to rate businesses during a service encounter. Their research initially led them to identify the following 10 dimensions, qualities, and characteristics that members (customers) look for and evaluate to determine whether they had a positive experience:

Tangibles	Reliability
Responsiveness	Competence
Courtesy	Credibility
Security	Access
Communication	Understanding the member/customer

A description of each dimension follows. Try to determine how the description applies to your club and any other business you conduct in or out of the club.

Tangibles

Tangibles relate to the appearance of the physical facility, the equipment, the staff, and any communication materials your club may use. It's whatever the members can get their hands on or their arms around. It also includes any other sensory experiences members will have in your club. How the club looks is very important because what members see is the first thing they notice about your club. This physical appearance is an important part of tangible service because many other parts of member service are intangible. The appearance of the club remains over time, but the services you provide vary and are used at the time they are offered. The member judges the appearance of the club and how the people who are providing the member services look as positive or negative. Remember, you only have one chance to make a first impression.

Have a nose for NEWS—what members need, expect, want, and what satisfies them.

Reliability

Reliability refers to your ability to perform and live up to your promises. When you promise to deliver something to a member in some form, you need to do just what you say you're going to do, and you must do it as dependably and accurately as possible. If a member calls you and you say you'll call back in 15 minutes, you must call back then and not in a day or two. If you're late in returning the call, the member will question your reliability. If you promise that your invoices to members will be error-free, do you make sure that you never send out an incorrect invoice? That's what the reliability dimension is all about. You do what you say you're going to do when you say you're going to do it, and you do it right the first time, every time.

Responsiveness

Responsiveness refers to your willingness to help members and the willingness of your employees to do the same. Do you provide prompt service when the member requires it? Do you resolve any problems or complaints quickly and to the member's total and complete satisfaction? If you schedule an appointment, are you there at the appropriate time? The answers to these questions determine how responsive you are to your members. Also, if you or your staff promise to deliver something, do you deliver exactly what you promised when you promised it? To improve responsiveness in your club, just respond to members' requests the way you want others to respond to your requests.

Competence

A competent service provider possesses the required skills and knowledge to perform the job well. You know exactly what you're supposed to do for the member and can do it without fumbling around, making mistakes, or delaying the transaction. You're also able to answer any questions the member may have. You build competence, and also confidence, by providing continuous, high-quality training and real-world learning experiences for yourself and your employees.

> *Superior member service requires you to be effective and to do the right things at the right time.*

I must emphasize one other point here. Many club owners provide skill-based training related to job performance and leave out the "softer skills" training such as communication, customer service, and interpersonal relations. Realize that these soft skills portray as much about a person's competence in our industry as extensive knowledge of personal training techniques does.

Courtesy

Courtesy is courtesy; it's as simple as that. It involves being polite, respectful, considerate, and friendly to members. As a club owner or department manager, these are also the behaviors you must exhibit to your employees. Be a role model and lead by example. When a member comes into your club, is there a friendly and positive atmosphere? Is the staff warm or rude to members? Do staff members stop what they're doing to serve a member in front of them? Do they focus their attention on the member in front of them and not on someone or something else?

You can think of many more questions and situations related to courtesy. If you need a standard to go by, just think about how you want to be treated and then be even more courteous than that to your members. Train your staff to call members by their last name (and use Mr. or Ms., as appropriate) and to always say "please" and "thank-you." Although this may seem like a minor point or intuitively obvious, you'd be surprised how many people forget the common courtesies as they go through their daily grind.

Credibility

Credibility is a function of your trustworthiness, honesty, and integrity. It also relates to your public image and reputation. Do you do what you say you're going to do? Are you consistent in your treatment of all members? If you offer a guarantee, do you live up to it? Can your members believe in and trust what you say? Remember that you and your employees are the club in the eyes and minds of your members. So if any of you lacks credibility for any reason, your club will also lack credibility. Members will begin to go elsewhere because no one wants to belong to a club that has people they can't trust.

Security

Security refers to safety, freedom from doubt, and the removal of risk factors. Members must feel secure when they join your club. They must first know that they are safe in coming to your club because the parking lot is well-lit at night, members aren't harassed by other members or staff, and members' valuables are safe in your locker rooms. There should be little to no risk for them to be a member at your club, either physically or financially, and they should get a physical, financial, and psychological return for their membership dues.

Access

Members want you, all your employees, and your customer service systems to be easily accessible. They want to be able to approach you whenever they need you, especially if you're the club owner or manager. You need to be available to them to provide great member service when they need it, not when it's convenient for you. If you're not available, then your competitors will be, and your members will become their members. Access refers to your staying open later in the evening, opening on weekends or holidays, opening earlier in the morning, and conducting club business when your member wants to meet with you. Accessibility means you make it easy and convenient for the member to be a member.

Communication

I believe that communication is the cause of all successes between people as well as the source of all disagreements and failures. When two people communicate effectively, things usually work out. When they don't communicate, problems occur.

Communication can make or break a member's perception of your club. How well do you keep members informed of what's going on in your club, in a language they can understand? How well do you listen to members? Do you explain things and make certain the member has a grasp of what you said? For example, have all the details of their membership contract been explained? Do they know exactly how their dues will be paid and when dues will be deducted from their checking or charge accounts? Are they aware that certain programs carry a separate charge in addition to their dues? If you and your staff communicate with members more effectively, you'll have more satisfied members who stay with you longer.

Understanding the Member/Customer

You've got to know your members intimately. Do whatever it takes to get information on the member, including likes, dislikes, hobbies, friends, needs, wants, expectations, birthday, family members, fitness goals, and anything else that might help you establish a relationship with that person. Where your regular members are concerned, make sure you recognize them when they come in and use their names correctly. Find out what their specific objectives are for coming to the club on a regular basis. Determine exactly what they want to achieve. Let them know that you understand them well and you still want to get to know them better. Sit down with all your members at least twice a year and have a personal discussion related to their fitness progress and their recommendations on how you can improve your service to them.

These are the original 10 dimensions of customer service that the researchers identified. Because members are customers, too, these descriptions and results are applicable to them also. Members use these dimensions to compare the service they expected to receive with the service they actually received to determine how satisfied they are in any given situation.

However, can you imagine trying to account for each or all of these 10 dimensions during every member service encounter? Further research supported the use of the first three categories and then created two groups for the last seven categories. Competence, courtesy, credibility, and security came under the new heading of assurance. *Assurance* is defined as the knowledge and courtesy of employees and their ability to convey trust and confidence. Access, communication, and understanding the member are now called empathy. *Empathy* refers to the caring, understanding, and individualized attention you provide your members. Reliability, tangibles, and responsiveness maintained the same definitions described earlier. This new organization created the five dimensions that members now use to act as a RATER of your club:

R= Reliability

A= Assurance

T= Tangibility

E= Empathy

R= Responsiveness

Members rate you continuously on these five dimensions. They may do it either consciously or subconsciously, but they definitely do it. They take a look at their needs, wants, and expectations, match their perception of these things with how well you're satisfying them directly and on each of these five dimensions, and then give you a subjective overall rating. This rating may or may not change over time. One thing you can be sure of is that this rating definitely determines how often and how much business they do with you and how long they stay as a member of your club. The question you must answer is how are you doing on these subjective member ratings? Once you know this, you must determine what you're going to do to improve your performance in each area.

Don't think that if you do well in two or three areas, it's sufficient. There's always another competitor who does well in all five areas, and this competitor will soon get your members. If members don't rate you high in all these areas, and if you haven't made either the financial or psychological switching costs too high for them or the proper adjustments in behavior to give the members what they want, they will go elsewhere. Sometimes, members will leave you because you were not giving them what they wanted in one area, not necessarily all five.

It doesn't take much to send a member elsewhere. Remember that 68 percent of people stopped doing business with a company because they didn't like the way they were treated. They had a bad encounter with a staff person, or they were ignored, or they just didn't like the tone of voice someone used. Who really knows what will upset a member? What we do know is that members leave, and sometimes, they leave in droves. When you consider that the average attrition rate for clubs hovers around 40 percent a year, there is plenty of room for improvement. This improvement will occur when you find out how the members rate you.

The key is to be proactive and learn exactly how members want to be treated by you and your staff. How will you know how members want to be treated? All you have to do is ask. After you ask and get the answers, then you can act accordingly to influence their rating process. You should also ask your staff to rate the club on these five dimensions. Then you can see whether there is a gap between what your staff perceives and what the members perceive. If there is, you must work diligently to close and eliminate those gaps.

Here's what you should do immediately: Evaluate your club on each of the five member rating areas and see where you stand. Develop a report card using grades like in school. Create your own scale if you want. Just come up with a way to objectively measure these criteria and quantify them. Then analyze your assessment. Develop a ratings index, a report card index, or a service index. What you call it doesn't matter as long as it gives you a benchmark against which you compare future evaluations. Make adjustments and improvements in areas where you are weak or lacking.

There are no right or wrong answers, just future success waiting for you if you do this, so I urge you to conduct this internal assessment of subjective perceptions with your members and staff as soon as possible. Don't become one of those clubs, or businesses in any industry for that matter, that had to close down because they just couldn't understand how their customers were rating them and why their customers were leaving them. The information is there. Just ask for it.

CHAPTER 4

Member Retention: The Backbone of Health Club Success

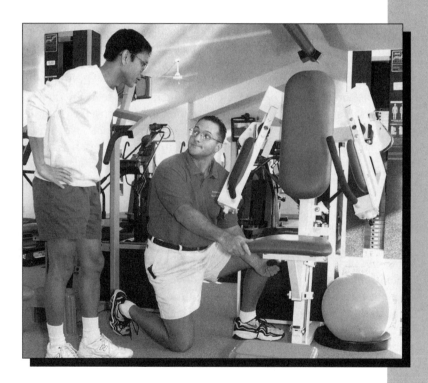

Many years ago, I was asked to be the evening sales manager for a chain of racquetball and health clubs in South Florida. I got this job because as a member of the club, I was responsible for bringing in more new members than the entire sales staff, except the day manager. The GM asked me if I'd help the club with sales during the evening and also assist with selling memberships at a new club the management was opening. I agreed, and little did I know that I was laying the foundation for many of my thoughts and my work in customer service and member retention.

Let me back up for a minute. I was a member of another club for two years. I was very close with the management and the staff. In fact, I had done some sales and service training for the staff, and the membership was steadily increasing. Yet to my surprise, as my membership was coming due, no one contacted me to renew. I was very disappointed. I figured this would be a great test to check out the true philosophy of the club: Were they more interested in new member sales or retaining current members?

It became obvious that no one was going to call me. My membership renewal was left up to me. I was responsible for keeping track of my due date and for initiating the resale. It was quite clear that the club's focus was on new sales instead of retention. When I realized this, I moved to the club mentioned previously. That's the reason I was able to sell so many memberships for my new club. Many of my friends came along with me just on my recommendation. So I made referral sales that showed up on the books as new sales.

While I was selling for the new facility, I asked the GM of my home club what was more important: Did the club managers want to keep their current members happy or were they more interested in constantly chasing and acquiring new members? I was told that the corporate office gave the managers a quota of a minimum of 100 new membership sales a month. I asked whether managers tracked attrition (and employee turnover), and they told me that it was an accepted part of the business, but they did not track it. They didn't have a real number for either factor.

Without knowing their attrition rate (or defection rate as it's currently called), they couldn't calculate the cost of losing a member, replacing a member, acquiring a new member, or retaining a current member. It's amazing how one little statistic can have such an impact on the business end of club operations. Yet many clubs today still don't know their attrition rate or the reasons for these defections. I know that the industry standard is somewhere around 40 or 50 percent, but that's not acceptable. It's way too high.

You need to know exactly how many members your club is losing each month, each quarter, and each year. You need to know what lost memberships cost you, as well as how much it costs you to acquire and retain one member. You also need to know what it costs in terms of time, energy, and money to replace the revenue a former member would have generated had he or she stayed with you.

By the way, the racquet and health club I was selling for did well for a while with new membership sales, but I just couldn't continue selling for the club when its focus was on getting new members instead of keeping current members happy. I knew then, as well as now, that in my training and consulting business, I must work very hard to satisfy and retain current customers to continue doing business with them. I also work hard to get new clients, but I don't neglect my current clients in the constant pursuit of new ones. So I stopped selling for that club. When my membership was due to expire, nobody even contacted me about renewing.

The message was clear. Membership retention was not an important issue to either club. Both of the clubs I've described to you went out of business. In talking with the members I knew from both facilities, I found out that the main reason they did not renew was that neither club paid attention to them. No one cared enough to even call or write that their memberships were expiring and ask them if they would like to renew. This complaint is right in line with a survey recently completed by IHRSA (International Health, Racquet and Sportsclub Association). The survey showed that 25 percent of members who left a club left because they were dissatisfied with the club. Data from the general business world shows that 68 percent of people stop being customers of a business because of the way they were treated (poor service, ignored by employees, and so on). These results underscore the need and importance for superior customer service focused on member retention.

> **How you treat members determines how long they'll stay around.**

Now I know today that you are very focused on membership retention. You probably track and calculate your attrition rate (as well as employee turnover, because member retention and employee retention are related). You may even know the cost of losing a member along with the lost opportunity revenues associated with a member defection. Hopefully, you've started calculating your member acquisition costs and the lifetime value of your members. All these numbers are important to your success and profitability in the club business.

Member Retention: It's Not Just About Programming

There is a big push in the industry to develop and implement a variety of programs that will enhance member retention. Things such as in-house clubs, at-home memberships, and free personal training all work toward improving membership retention—we think; we hope. Although chapter 12 describes 25 member retention programs and activities that work for clubs, member retention is not about programming.

It's about a philosophy of doing business.

It's about a corporate culture of focusing on your members (customers).

It's about the financial impact of defection versus retention.

It's about all these things and more.

Since 1990, I've informally asked over 100 club owners and sales managers/ membership directors a year what they are doing to keep members. Over 90 percent of the people tell me they are developing and implementing "creative member retention programs (whatever that means)." Think about it. What's the difference between a membership sales program (discounts, two-fers, family packages, and so on) that changes each month and a membership retention program that changes each month? In the minds of your members, there is no difference. It's a flavor-of-the-month perception. "If this one doesn't work for me," the member thinks, "I'll wait for the next one. Something is bound to come along that I'll like. If it doesn't, I'll just sign up somewhere else for a better deal or lower price."

Member retention is not about programs, no matter how creative your programs are. I talked with one membership director whose club chain is well-known for innovative and creative retention programs. When we talked more in depth, he told me that the chainwide attrition rate exceeds 50 percent. Can you imagine? The chain is well-known in the industry for its retention programs, yet these same retention programs don't work well for the chain. What are we to make of this?

The answer is the same thing all over again. Member retention is not about programs. It's not about doing things at a point in time to try to increase retention and slow the attrition rate. What it is about is developing an ongoing philosophy and approach to club operations that focuses on retaining members, increasing their loyalty, and developing a win-win partnership with them.

A New Paradigm of Thought for Clubs: Be Member-Oriented Rather Than Profit-Oriented

The approach you must now take is to focus more on your members and their needs and expectations than you do on your profit. When you serve members well and provide them with value, they will provide you with increased profits. You must become truly member-oriented if you want to increase your member retention rates. This section gives you some ways to become more member-oriented.

Get to know your members as well as they know themselves. Use the technology in your front desk systems to keep track of member-related information. Use your staff as well: Have your staff talk to members, get to know them personally, and then share this information with the rest of the staff. The more you know about your members and the more you can treat them as individuals, the better your chances are of retaining them over time.

As you and your members and staff learn more about each other, you become partners in the club experience. I'm not suggesting that you bring members into your club business financially; I am suggesting that you work with them to make sure their entire membership experience is positive. Work hard to build up trust with your members, because that is a major perceptual basis for retention and loyalty. Be honest with them and respect them. Find out what they need, want, and expect from you, and then give it to them. Do whatever it takes to help them get the fitness results they joined for and the psychological results they come back for. As partners, your goal is to make each of your lives better. Help them win!

When members join your club, they have every intention of staying with you over the long term; they don't want to throw their money away. Keeping this fact in mind should help you work to keep your members for life. Understand that when they buy your product (the membership), they want to receive value for their payment: they want their workouts to be of superior quality, they want to fully understand and then achieve the benefits you promised during the sale, and they want you to be reliable. In other words, they want the club to be there and open when they want to work out. They also want to receive a high level of service that respects them as individuals. Every experience and encounter with your club should be positive and provide an additional setting for both of you to learn more about each other.

When you invest this much time in a person, you tend to prefer to stay with that person longer. This tendency works for you trying to keep the member and for the member wanting to stay with your club. You must continue to build on this relationship in order to retain the member. Make sure you and your staff are accessible when members need you. You must also be accountable for your service efforts—never pass off the responsibility for service to someone else. Whoever meets the member owns that encounter, and each individual encounter can make or break your relationship. Therefore, all staff members must be committed to providing excellent service 100 percent of the time. They must do whatever it takes to serve, satisfy, and retain members.

If this level of service seems extremely difficult to provide, it is, but it's essential to the success of your club. If you're not willing to go to these lengths, I know many clubs that are. They will gladly take your members. The only way to prevent defection and keep members for life is to work hard at building solid member relationships. Think back to your service philosophy. Is it member-friendly? Is it designed to include members in your club's operation? Is it designed to make members feel at home in your club? Does it guarantee your service? Does it guarantee that your service systems are easily accessible and member-friendly? Does it guarantee that your employees are fully empowered to serve members?

Consider these important issues as you focus on member retention. You must always remember that service is the start of retention. If the beginning of the experience is bad for the member, you'll always be in a catch-up mode, and that's no way to run a business. Be proactive with your members and build your relationships with them. Interact with them as often as possible to learn as much as you can about them. Don't be like the club owner I once knew who sat in his office and looked out through his glass window at the workout floor, but never came out to meet the members. His philosophy was that he was giving them a place to work out; he didn't have to be their friend. He is no longer a club owner, but you could have guessed that.

Deliver on your promises and meet or exceed the expectations of your members. Don't promise anything you can't deliver. If they want something from you and you can't do it for them, tell them immediately. They will appreciate your honesty. If they want something customized from you, and you can do this for them, do it! They will appreciate your effort. In fact, the more you can customize and individualize programs and services for members, the greater the chances are that they will stay with you over the long term. The fact that you're treating them as individuals will make them want to stay with you even more.

If you make a mistake, recover from it and make sure the member is satisfied with your recovery. Train your staff to know their jobs and to be friendly, polite, courteous, and service-oriented. Empower them to serve the members whenever and wherever service is needed. Invest in your staff and your members, and they will invest in you. This exchange is what true member orientation is about. The result is that superior service will help you keep your members for life.

The Importance of Customer Service and Member Retention to Club Business Success

Member retention begins with superior customer service. Customer service is the critical factor for succeeding in the health-and-fitness club business today. You must provide customer service that is far superior to that offered by your competitors in order for you to attract and keep members who remain loyal and help you make a profit. Remember that customer retention and lowered customer acquisition costs, not new customer acquisition, result in the greatest profit.

Much of customer service and customer retention comes down to simple common sense. Common sense customer service encompasses everything you and your employees do to satisfy members. You give them what they want and make sure they're happy. If you just manage complaints, offer refunds, or smile at members, you are only providing a small part of excellent customer service. Customer service also means going out of your way for the member, doing everything possible to satisfy the member, and making decisions that benefit the member, sometimes even at the expense of the club. (When this situation occurs, consider the future potential of that member's business with you.) The goal of customer service is not only to satisfy the member, but also to make sure that member stays around for a long time. In other words, the goal of customer (member) service is member retention.

The Importance of Customer Service

How important is customer service to the success of your club? It can make or break you. Suppose you and your competitors are selling memberships at basically the same price. You both have similar equipment, well-trained staff, and a beautiful facility. The clubs' locations are easy to access, and the hours of operation are just what the members want. You have nothing physical to greatly differentiate your club from your competitors, so what will make members join your club instead of your competitors' clubs?

The answer is very simple. The determining factor is the level and quality of customer service you provide. All things being equal, people will join a club that treats them like first-class citizens. If you had your choice, and price was not an issue, would you stay at a Ritz-Carlton or a Motel 6? Would you drive a Lexus or a Chevy, based on what you know about the personal service you receive from each dealership? Would you go to the club where everyone knows your name or where they couldn't care less about you?

Everyone in your club is a customer service representative.

The answer, again, is very simple and obvious. You go where you receive the best service. (Note also that people will pay for service.) What do I mean by service? It's the way you and your employees treat members. It's the way you answer the telephone and listen to member requests for information on your programs and services. It's how your club and the equipment look, because appearance is a major determinant of service perceptions. It's how well you treat the members after they become members, a factor which could be the most important part of your service efforts leading to member retention. Ask yourself this question: Do you treat members as part of your family or do they just become a number after they join? (One of the top three complaints members have about clubs is that they become just a number and lose their identity.)

All these things relate to customer service and the impression members have of you. If these impressions and perceptions are positive, they not only will do business with you, they also will continue to do business with you. They will stay with you over time and continue to become more and more profitable for your club. On the other hand, if members have negative perceptions of the service they receive, or if you have done something to upset members, you can be sure they will go down the street to one of your competitors. They may do this while still maintaining their membership with you until it expires, or they may wait until it expires and then leave you. In either case, you've lost members you did not have to lose to a competitor. There are things you can do to prevent them from walking out. Remember that your goal in providing great customer service is to create members for life.

The Payoff of Superior Customer Service

Several years ago, you couldn't pay some clubs to train their employees to provide good customer service. Either clubs did not view customer service as important, or they didn't think the training was important, or they didn't think the employees warranted training beyond specific job skills. Some businesses that I've worked with, mostly outside the fitness industry, felt that customers would come in, buy something, use it, and eventually leave the business anyway, so it didn't matter whether you were nice to them.

Can you believe that mind-set in today's competitive environment? Can you believe that some clubs still think this way, even with attrition rates as high as 70 to 80 percent? How do I know these clubs exist? I talk to them and listen to what they say. It amazes me that any club owner can think more in terms of member acquisition or member replacement instead of member retention, but some do. As I've said before, when it comes right down to it, all of today's clubs are basically the same bricks and mortar. How you treat the members determines how long they'll stay around.

Customer service pays, and it does not cost you anything. Yes, you may have to spend some dollars up front in training programs for your staff, and there may be some other costs involved in revamping or revising your service delivery systems within your club. You may also have to invest in the development of retention and loyalty management programs as a business philosophy. But in the long run, customer service always pays off.

The way it pays off the most is in long-term member retention. Keeping members and doing business with them repeatedly is much less expensive and much more profitable than trying to find new members all the time. Always remember that it costs you much more to acquire a new member than it does to retain a current member.

Some Examples of the Dollar Value of Customer Service

I've already talked about the dollar value of customer service in chapter 1. However, it's so important that I'm repeating similar examples here.

Some businesses and clubs know the cost of acquiring a new customer; others do not have a clue what new customer acquisition costs them. You need to know this cost before you can calculate the financial benefits of member retention for your club. Those clubs that know what it costs to acquire a new member are bending over backward to keep the members they have happy. The many club owners who are not even aware of the extraordinary costs of losing a customer just figure that if someone doesn't renew their membership one day, another person will buy one the next. Wrong!

There are three things you must know about the payoff for providing excellent customer service that leads to long-term member retention. Research in the general business field estimates that it costs five to six times more to acquire a new customer than it does to do business with a current or former customer. Some research has even said that it costs 10 times more to get a new customer. In either case, getting new customers is quite expensive. Suppose you calculate the cost of acquiring a new member and it is $500. Then you figure out that it only costs you about $100 to do business (work to retain) with a current member. That's a $400 savings that becomes profit in your club when you retain members instead of replace them.

Second, whenever you lose members, there are costs associated with replacing them, and you lose the revenue their membership would have provided during the replacement period. There is also something called lost opportunity revenue, which is all the potential money you could have made from those members if you kept them loyal and they continued to purchase from you over an extended period of time. These purchases include items from your pro shop, non-dues revenue programs, additional personal training, and anything else in addition to their membership dues.

The third thing is the cost of negative word of mouth. Whenever you lose a member, it is usually because that member had a bad experience with you. Research from the general business world shows that you can control between 96 and 99 percent of the reasons people stop doing business with you, depending on the type of business you have. So if your customer service is excellent, you should only lose a small number of members. But if you dissatisfy even one member, that person may tell up to 20 people about the bad service they received. The odds are good that these 20 people will not do business with you at all. If they don't join because of negative word of mouth, which could have been prevented by excellent customer service, then you're losing a great deal of money. Calculate that lost opportunity revenue over a 3-, 5-, or 10-year period. If that's not mind-boggling enough, consider the geometric progression of 20 people telling 20 people telling another 20 people not to join your club because you provide bad service to the members.

Can you really afford to have all these people not join your club because of bad service? Can you really afford to lose even one member because of bad service? Add the costs of these three reasons together, and you get a pretty good idea of how valuable and profitable it is to retain members for a long time by providing superior customer service. It's easy to see how very costly it is if you provide poor service. With this cost in mind, it's not whether you can afford to train your staff to provide excellent customer service, it's can you afford not to?

You must focus your entire club operation around serving, satisfying, and retaining members. Consider the payoff in money earned or saved by keeping your members against what it costs you to replace them when you lose them. To put it very simply, customer service, member satisfaction, and long-term member retention are vitally important to your success in every aspect of the club business. Your newfound focus on retention will allow you to create a more profitable club environment.

Three New Ways to Use Member Retention to Grow Your Club Business

Take a look at your club. What is the level of commitment from owners, managers, and supervisors, as well as staff, to doing whatever it takes to satisfy your members? What about your workout guarantees—the results you promise members? Do you make the purchase of your membership risk-free beyond the three-day cooling-off period? Who is responsible for delivering service to the members? Is it a membership service department, your sales department, or everyone who comes in contact with members? If it's not the latter, then you're in trouble. Remember that everyone in your club is a service representative. This concept is important, so let me repeat it. Everyone in your club is a customer service representative.

Because many clubs are doing and saying the same things and making the same offers, you need to create a way to differentiate your club from your competitors. Again, it's not going to be in the retention programs that you offer. Your competitors can provide the same programs. The differentiating factor will be in how you operate your club. When you focus on member retention from the beginning, you instill a completely different mind-set and culture in your club. One key to instilling this member retention culture is to embrace the concepts of loyalty management, defection management, and revenue management. Although these three concepts have nothing to do with delivering member service directly, they have everything to do with satisfying members, increasing member retention, and creating high member loyalty.

Loyalty Management

We'll talk more about loyalty later in the book. For now, understand that there is a tremendous difference between a satisfied member and a loyal member. Satisfied members may not be loyal. I know that sounds crazy, but satisfaction, retention, and loyalty mean different things. Satisfied members are happy with the service you provide and the value they receive for their money. A satisfied member may be one who does not complain or just has nothing negative to say about your club. Such members may be retainable because you haven't done anything to send them away.

Although they are satisfied and retainable, they may not be loyal. They may buy from you and also buy from your competitors, such as holding memberships in both your club and a YMCA. Or they may purchase clothes in your pro shop but purchase nutritional supplements in a health food store instead of from you. In this case, they are satisfied, but they are not totally loyal. You don't have the share of member (or share of wallet) that you really want. They are spending money elsewhere that could be spent with you. So in addition to member satisfaction and retention, another goal of your business is to increase your share of the member's wallet, which means increasing his or her loyalty to your club.

Take a poll of your members. How loyal are they? Do they buy everything from you, or do they split up their purchases? Check your database, and do an analysis of member expenditures. Then ask them where else they are spending their money. This information will give you an indication of their loyalty and your share of their wallet.

MEMBER RETENTION IS ABOUT:

A philosophy of doing business.

A corporate culture of focusing on your members (customers).

The financial impact of defection versus retention.

All these things and more.

Do you do any frequency marketing programs? An example of such a program is a punch card in an ice cream store. After 10 purchases, you get a free cone. Many stores and businesses do this or something like it. Are you doing something similar? If you are, go back and review your frequency marketing programs along with your reward and recognition programs for members. Who has participated in them? How effective have they been in attracting and keeping members? Have they generated incremental revenues for your club?

All this activity is part of loyalty management. You need to go beyond satisfaction to create advocates, apostles, and loyal followers. Here are some things you can do to build loyalty:

1. Identify who your right members are. (They are the most profitable and require the least amount of service.)

2. Find out exactly what they need, want, and expect from you.

3. Determine their desired level of service.

4. Give them more than they ask for and expect.

5. Beg them for feedback so you can improve.

6. Implement their feedback suggestions.

7. Build a personal and psychologically rewarding relationship with them.

8. Provide them with recognition and reward programs.

9. Show them you appreciate their loyalty by giving them preferential treatment.

10. Help them improve their lives or even grow their businesses.

These are some of the best ways you can manage loyalty in your club and with your members. Do the same things for your employees, so they will provide better member service, stay loyal to you, and help your members become more loyal at the same time.

Defection Management

The number one problem for any club is losing members. Although our industry calls it attrition, the official business term is customer defections. Members leave your business, for one reason or another, and usually go to a competitor. Even if they don't join another club, you have lost their membership fees and any other revenues they would have generated. You need to learn why members are leaving your club. You need to survey them, interview them, or somehow get them to tell you their reasons for leaving. Then, you must categorize these reasons to determine your areas for improvement. You must manage these defections, or you run the risk of losing your club.

You must engage in the following 10 activities to effectively manage the defections from your club.

1. Provide great customer service to all members at all times.

2. Keep track of how many members leave your business and when they go.

3. More specifically, determine how many members from a particular time period leave and when.

4. Contact these members to identify the reasons for their defections and identify the appropriate defection patterns.

5. Calculate your defection rate, first as a percentage and then as a fraction.

6. Flip the fraction to get your retention rate.

7. Compare the defecting members with your share of customer percentage to see if these defectors are in the bottom 20 percent of your profit contributors, the middle, or the top 20 percent. If they are in the bottom 20 percent, don't worry about them; they may cost more to keep than to let go. If they are that unprofitable, send them to a competitor club.

8. Go after the top 20 percent of your defectors and find out what you must do to get them back.

9. Develop specialty return programs and other inducements to win back your members.

10. Analyze your defection patterns and institute programs to overcome them.

Defection management or its twin, retention management, is essential for your success. You must simultaneously stop the flow of people leaving your club while improving the areas of service that are causing them to leave. Most club owners will tell you that their attrition (defection) rate is around 40 to 50 percent annually, so retention management is a critical success factor. It's a difficult task, but one that every club owner must do in order to remain successful. As you can see, retention management is not just about programming any more.

Revenue Management (Market Value Pricing)

The revenue management or market value pricing (MVP) concept may be new to some, and not to others. MVP is basically a variable pricing strategy. It works like this: When you've completed your loyalty management and defection analysis processes, you will know exactly who your best members are. You should also know how much they buy from you, when they buy, their preferential times of purchase, and other important specific pieces of information that are a result of your close relationship with these members.

Now you must ask these members how much more they would appreciate the value you're providing. Tell them that you'll customize your product or service even more for them if they'd be willing to pay a slightly higher price. Most of your best members won't mind paying the additional money for continued and better service. Even if a few people mind, they'll realize that the value you provide far exceeds the costs they incur by purchasing from you. That's because you're providing them with customized programs and services. So you'll even get to keep some of your dissenters as members.

You're already familiar with this concept of market value pricing. Airlines do it all the time. The closer you buy a ticket to your departure time, the more it costs you. Health clubs do it also with their different levels of membership based on usage and time of day. Movie theaters also manage their revenues this way, charging less for shows earlier in the day when supposedly fewer people can attend. Even a hair salon can conduct business with a market value pricing approach by having those people who absolutely must come on weekends pay higher prices.

Look around your club and determine ways to manage your revenues. Using the MVP concept will increase your revenues and contribute to your profitability. Your best members will not mind paying more for the higher level of service they receive. You use MVP anyway with your more expensive membership levels and what they include over a basic membership. Now you have to create an operating model to base these price differences on service and improving retention and use a variety of loyalty management techniques to keep members for life.

> **Get to know your members as well as they know themselves.**

There you have three distinct and already proven ways you can grow your business. Although they are not directly a form of customer service, they are directly related to delivering high-quality customer service to get and retain members for life. It is up to you to figure out exactly how to implement these management techniques into your club business.

Remember, that while other clubs are spending wildly to achieve higher and higher levels of market share, you can be working diligently and inexpensively to increase your level of customer/member wallet share. Would you rather have a lot of members buying small amounts from you once or once in a while, or would you rather have a select group of members buying large amounts from you more often? Also, remember that the longer members stay with you, the more profitable those members become for you. Add to their own purchases the referrals they generate for your club, as well as the positive word-of-mouth marketing they do for you. To me, customer/member share is the clear winner over market share. That's why I always say that member retention is the backbone of success in the club industry. What do you think?

part two

Customer Service Skills

CHAPTER 5

The Telephone Is Your Member Service Lifeline

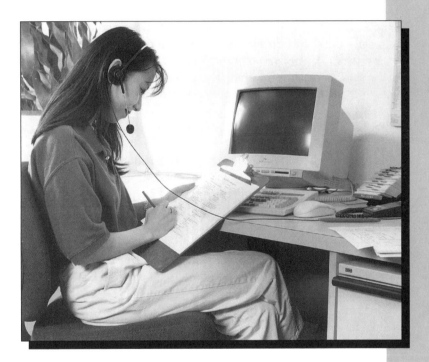

A couple of years ago, a client asked me to shop her club and her competitors by telephone. She wanted to know how well her staff responded to telephone inquiries, how they handled membership and pricing questions, and how they communicated with the caller. She also wanted to compare the performance of her staff with those of competitor clubs. So she had me call around as a prospective member. You know the drill. You've been shopped by your competitors over the phone dozens of times every year. The only difference between the secret shop and what I was doing was that I was conducting legitimate research for a client to improve her service to her members.

I made nine calls in all. Six were to competitors, and three were to her club at different times with different requests. On three of the calls to competitor clubs, I was put on hold by the person answering the phone for over 60 seconds. When that person returned and I explained the nature of my request, two of them told me they couldn't help me and that a salesperson would have to call me back. The third transferred me to a salesperson who told me he was too busy at the time doing paperwork. He asked me to leave my number, and he'd call back. I told him I'd call back when I had the chance.

On the other three calls to competitors, I was greeted very nicely on the phone, and that person answered all my questions about the location, the equipment, the size of the facility, the staffing ratios, the number of personal trainers, the number of aerobics and other classes, the philosophy of the club, and the future plans for the club. Two of the people quoted me membership prices over the phone; the third person asked me to come in for a tour.

When I called my client's club, the first occasion was to inquire about membership. I was put on hold, and then, after what seemed like an eternity, I was told that there were no membership sales directors available to talk to me. Could I please call back? The second call asked about the equipment, the staff, their credentials and training, and the classes. These questions were all answered to my satisfaction. My third call had me playing the role of an upset member who was complaining that my account was being double-billed through EFT (electronic funds transfer). I was so irate that the poor person answering the phone couldn't get a word in edgewise. She got flustered and told me to hold on while she got the owner. When my client came on the line, I told her it was me and said I'd be in to discuss my findings shortly.

What can we learn from this telephone research? We learn that all your staff members must be able to handle any type of phone inquiry that comes in. It is essential for everyone to have most, if not all, the answers because people will not stay on hold very long, nor will they accept incompetent (as they perceive it) staff members. Your role and goal is to emphasize the importance of the telephone to the success of your club.

The telephone is the heart and soul of every club when it comes to member service. Just like I did in the previous examples, people will call you to find out where you are located, to check on membership availability and pricing, to learn your hours of operation, to ask questions, to register complaints, and just to talk. Much of your club's success is dependent on how well you and your employees handle the phone. This issue may seem trivial to you because you assume effective telephone skills are a given. Unfortunately, they're not a given. Phone skills are so bad across so many different industries that several training companies base their entire curriculum on telephone skills training.

Even with knowing these programs are available, and even with knowing that a majority of first contacts with clubs come through the phone, we still let bad service on the telephone happen.

You call a club, or any company for that matter, and the phone rings and rings and no one picks up, not even an answering machine. When the phone is finally answered, the person puts you on hold without ever giving you a chance to state the reason for your call. Or you call a company, and an automatic call distribution system picks up and tells you your options; then when you press your option, you get even more options. You press your option again, and there's nobody to answer the call personally. Or you call someplace, and a person answers the phone with "Yeah, whadda ya want?" Or you call a club, and a person answers "Who's this?"

It's amazing that in this day and age, with so much material being produced and published on the importance of customer service and retention, companies still allow their employees to display atrocious telephone skills. What makes it even worse is when you, as a member, walk into the club and the receptionist is too busy handling a personal call to even acknowledge your entrance. Does this happen in your club? Even if it never happens, let this be an instructive example of what not to do and what you should never allow to happen.

Call your own club to determine how well your employees answer the phone. Listen with extra care from two perspectives: as the manager/owner and as a member. It's amazing what you'll learn when you frame your perceptions from someone else's position. You may also want to have someone else call your club and go through a problem scenario to see how well your staff handles the situation on the phone. This exercise alone could provide you with invaluable feedback. If you've never done either or both of these things, you should. You'll gain a world of insight into the effect the phone is having on your club and the effect your staff is having on the phone.

The Beginnings of Superior Telephone Member Service

The beginning of great member service starts when the phone rings. Every time that phone rings, it's an opportunity for you to make a sale or to provide a value-added service that psychologically links the member to you for a longer period of time. To reinforce this idea, in some training sessions, I have the staff imagine that the ringing phone is a cash register bell. This image brings home the financial importance of relating to the caller every time the phone rings. It doesn't matter whether the caller is a current member, a former one, or a prospective member. Whoever is calling is calling for a reason, and you or your staff can create the right or the wrong atmosphere and perceptions of your club just by how well you handle the phone call.

Begin by establishing a set of standards related to telephone behavior. The first standard is that no one answers the phone without knowing how all the features work. That's right. You must train everyone on your staff, even part-timers, on how the phones work. It's not fair to practice on the caller, nor is it quality service to say "I'll try to transfer you, but I don't know exactly how to use this phone. If I lose you, call back, and I'll find someone who can get you to the right person." This scene plays out time and again in clubs and other businesses around the world. It's not the caller's responsibility to call back or to wait for you to learn how the phone works. Do that before you even get near a phone in your club.

Another standard may be the tone of voice that people use when they answer the phone. Your smile comes across loud and clear on the phone. It's essential that everyone is positive and promotes the great lifestyle of fitness, especially at your club. I worked with one club owner who couldn't figure out why members were registering so many complaints about the way the phone was answered. The receptionist in question was answering the phone using the script that was developed; she knew how to use the phone, and she was pleasant to talk to face-to-face. The problem was that she spoke in a monotone voice on the phone and never generated any enthusiasm. So when someone called, that person was immediately brought down instead of lifted up because of her voice. Make sure everyone uses an upbeat tone of voice. You can even put a sticker on the phone that says, "Smile! The boss is calling."

> **The telephone is the heart and soul of every club when it comes to member service.**

Another standard, and one that is more typical, is that the phone must be answered by the third ring. I suggest three rings for two reasons. First, people don't like to be kept waiting, and answering the phone by the third ring is fairly prompt. Two rings would be better. Is one ring the best? I don't know. How anxious are you to get to the phone? Second, the third ring on your end of the line can actually be the fourth ring on their end. I'm sure you've made calls where the other person picked it up and said it didn't even ring, and you heard it ring once or even twice on your end. So it's entirely possible that your third ring is the fourth or fifth ring in the customer's ear.

Waiting while the phone is ringing can be annoying, especially in this day and age. Today, we expect a person, an answering machine, or voice mail to pick up the phone after a set number of rings. When the phone just keeps ringing, it gets terribly annoying to the caller. When you realize that a person who is waiting for anything, such as a phone to be answered or a line to move forward, psychologically doubles their waiting time, you know why it's so important to answer the phone as quickly as possible. Phone response time is easy to measure because you can ask members how often the phone was answered by the third ring and use their answers to develop improvement strategies.

After you've established the three-ring standard, you need establish a simple phone greeting that everyone must use. The staff should speak the greeting as you establish it, but remember that everyone must be able to inject his or her own personality into answering and speaking on the phone. The purpose for standardizing the phone greeting is so that callers will come to expect a high level of professionalism, courtesy, and member service from you and your staff every time they call. When you link the phone greeting with the high level of service the members receive on the phone and when they come into the club, they become conditioned. Every time they call, your personalized and standardized greeting will trigger positive thoughts and feelings and reinforce why they should be and are members in your club. When your telephone greeting makes them feel good, they'll definitely consider doing more business with you. All this simply because of the way you answer the phone.

Your telephone answering script for all employees should be something like this: When the phone rings, the person answering it takes a deep breath, smiles, gets ready to be positive (all this takes microseconds), and then picks up the phone and says "Hello, (or good morning, good afternoon, and so on), ABC Fitness Center. This is (your name). How may I help you?" By asking how you may help the caller, you've invited that person into a friendly conversation. When you ask "May I help you?", you've given the caller the opportunity to say no. But by asking how, you're opening the door for callers to give you more information. Remember, the only way you can determine what a member needs and how you can best satisfy those needs is to ask questions.

To summarize, great telephone member service begins when you establish a set of telephone standards. Train yourself and your staff in how the phone system works. Have everyone answer the phone within three rings. When you or a staff member answer the phone, use an upbeat tone of voice and greet the caller, identify your club, identify yourself, and ask "How may I help you?" The caller then begins a dialogue with you where the caller speaks more often and you listen. The only time you talk more than the caller is when you're responding to one of his or her questions.

The concept of telephone dialogue is critical to your success. Dialogue means a two-way conversation between you and the caller. A monologue is a one-way conversation, and it can get boring for the listener. That's especially true if the listener is the caller, and you start to monopolize the conversation. Too often, club employees get involved with monologues where they're telling the member everything they think the member wants to hear or know. The stimulus can be a question the caller asked, or sometimes it's just the fact that the staff person answered the phone and began talking. If the club person would just keep quiet for a few minutes and let the caller/member talk, she would learn a great deal about why that person called in the first place.

During a telephone dialogue, you must remember that the member cannot see you. So you've got to impart certain feelings to that member in a variety of ways. Begin with a smile. The muscles that cause your face to smile have a positive effect on the muscles that help you speak, and your smile definitely comes through on the telephone. Just ask anyone who is on the other end. Members can tell whether you're smiling and happy to speak with them or whether it's a chore. When you smile while talking on the phone, both you and the person on the other end of the line will be more relaxed, and the conversation will take on a more personal and friendly tone.

Next, monitor your tone of voice. Speak in a pleasant manner so that the tone conveys the message of your words. Don't tell the caller you're happy to speak with them or help them when your tone of voice is rushed or stressed. The caller will pick up any incongruity in your speech, and you'll have a hard time communicating. You may have the best of intentions, but your underlying message will be the exact opposite of your words.

If you don't believe this, think about a time when you've been in a conversation or argument with someone close to you. They say something that upsets you. It's no big deal to them what they said, but you're visibly upset. They ask you why you're upset because they don't perceive they've said anything that could hurt your feelings. You say that it's not what they said but how they said it. The key here is how they said it, which relates primarily to their tone of voice.

Think of a club situation where a member is asking a staff person for information. Unfortunately, the member caught the staff person as he or she was about to do something else or leave work for the day. During the conversation, the staff person keeps looking around, paying only partial attention to the member. Although the staff person may be saying he or she wants to help the member, his or her actions betray what's being said. The how doesn't match the what.

How you say something conveys more meaning than what you say. Communications research shows us that how you say something accounts for 93 percent of the meaning of your message; only 7 percent is accounted for by what you say. So when you speak with someone over the phone, keep your tone upbeat and positive. Concentrate on how you're saying what you're saying. Match the how with the what. Don't let your speech convey annoyance, boredom, impatience, or a lack of interest in what the member is saying. If you do, that member will just hang up and never call back, and the next call he or she makes will be to your competitor.

The next important thing for you to do is use words and sentences the caller can understand. Now is not the time to show off how smart you are by using technical terms, industry jargon, acronyms, or big words. It does you no good if a prospective member calls to inquire about your club's programs, services, and equipment, and your staff member starts talking about $\dot{V}O_2$max, FEV, biomarkers, or any other inside terms or phrases.

Speak so the caller understands you. Don't mumble. Speak clearly and enunciate your words, especially if there are regional accent differences. Speak slowly but not so slowly that you become boring. If there are accent differences, you should still speak in your normal voice. There is no reason to speak louder just because you're from one part of the country and the caller is from another. Increasing the volume of your voice will not help the listener understand you any better on the phone.

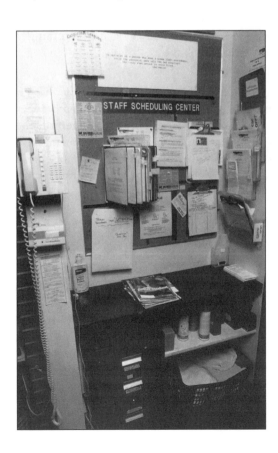

Listen to everything the member has to say. Listening becomes even more important during telephone member service because you can't see the caller's reactions and responses to your words. So you must listen for the words and the hidden meanings between the words. I'll discuss listening skills in greater detail later in the book.

If you just pay attention to these few suggestions, your telephone member service skills will increase dramatically. The next section gives several more ideas to help you provide superior telephone member service.

10 More Great Telephone Member Service Tips

You already know how important it is to answer the phone promptly, greet the caller correctly, and speak in an ordinary conversation voice. It is just as important to do the following to make a good impression on your caller:

1. **Always have a pad and pencil/pen near the phone**. A member who calls to give you some information will be annoyed if you tell him or her to wait while you find something to write with and something to write on. If the paper and pen are near the phone at all times, you can begin taking notes as soon as you answer the call.

2. If you are computerized (and you already know that I believe you must be in order to provide continuous, high-quality member service), **access the member's record as soon as he identifies himself on the call.** This way, you have all the information you need about the member (who he is, membership history, workout history, past purchase history, series of complaints, requests, and needs, and so on) right there in front of you. Plus, you can take notes right in the program to update the record.

A member database does wonders for any business, and it will do the same for your club. Unfortunately, as I've informally surveyed club owners over the years, I can tell you that over 85 percent of the clubs are not using their computer technology to its fullest capacity. You have at your disposal the technology and the techniques to establish and solidify long-term member relationships. Yet most clubs use the front desk system as a high-powered check-in system instead of all that it is capable of. It's like those people who buy the expensive organizers with the leather covers. There is so much potential in using the system, but they use it as an expensive calendar instead of a true planner/organizer. The same goes for computer systems and technology in clubs—they are usually not used to their fullest extent.

In my own business, when customers from long ago call me up to discuss something, and they ask if I remember what we talked about last year, or two years ago, they're amazed at how accurate my memory is. I can tell them what we talked about, when we talked about it, and what the outcome of our conversation was. I can even tell them the date and time we talked. Although this seems like an amazing memory trick, in reality, all I'm doing is reading them the notes from my customer database. It doesn't matter what type of club you're in. A member database is crucial to your success as an operator and a member service provider. The proper and comprehensive use of your technology is also critical.

3. **Own the calls you answer**. If the call is an information request or a problem to be resolved, try to take care of it. Members appreciate a club where they can call and the first person they speak to can help them. Members, and people calling any business, resent being transferred and having to repeatedly explain why they called, especially when they believe the person who answered the phone could have handled the call.

4. **Address the caller properly**. If the member gives you her name, use it. Ask if you can call her by her first name or if she prefers you use her last name. Use her name as often as you can during the conversation to establish rapport. Just make sure that you say the name properly. Nothing can ruin a conversation faster than a staff person saying the caller's name incorrectly.

5. **When you have to transfer a member, bridge the call with the member and with the person who'll be receiving the call from you.** If you have to transfer a member to another staff person, do the following. First, ask the member if they would mind being put on hold while you transfer the call to someone else who can help them more effectively. When they give you permission to put them on hold, transfer the call and tell the person who'll be receiving the call exactly what the member told you. There's nothing more irritating for a member than to keep being transferred around in a club and having to repeat the same story over and over again. The member should tell the story once, and you should be able to communicate that situation to the staff member who will handle the situation. Then the person who takes the call from you should do whatever it takes to help serve and satisfy the member.

You may already know that there is telephone software that integrates with computers to display the member's record on the screen of the person to whom the call is transferred. I'm not saying that your club should invest in this technology just yet. I am saying that you should use the model and provide the information to the second staff person so the calling member does not have to repeat the reason for the call.

If you have to put a member on hold for any other reason, ask that member's permission first, as you would if you were transferring the call. If you do put a member on hold, make sure you come back to the phone every 30 to 60 seconds to tell the member how much longer he or she will be on hold.

Customers on hold perceptually double or triple the actual waiting time. When their wait is perceived as too long, you get back on the line with an annoyed or irate member.

6. When you complete the conversation, **thank the member for calling and gently hang up the receiver.** Don't slam it down, and don't start talking to someone else before the receiver is hung up. This tip is especially important if you use a speaker phone. (Also, you should never pick up a phone while you're in the middle of a conversation with another person, while you're laughing, or while you're coughing. The caller hears all these things, and they don't portray a positive service image.) Sometimes, staff people make a comment about a member to another staff member when they believe the phone is on the hook or the speaker is off. Unfortunately, this is not always the case, and the member hears the remark. Before you or anyone else says anything about a just-completed call, make sure the receiver is on the hook, and the speaker is off.

7. **If a member puts you on hold, wait on the line until he comes back to you.** It sends a poor message and provides a bad impression about your club if, while a member has you on hold, you put him on hold without asking his permission while you attend to something else.

8. Whether members call you or you call them, **always be enthusiastic, friendly, and positive.** Your attitude and mood will be contagious, and the member will enjoy doing business with such a positive person. Plus, if this is a prospective member's first contact with your club, think of the wonderful and positive first impression you just made. Members will carry that impression with them for a long time.

9. **Follow up on the phone.** When someone calls you with a request, regardless of the nature of the request, call that person back in a day or two to make sure she is satisfied with how you handled the call. Even if the call was for membership information, you should capture the essential data of name, address, and phone number for your database. Then, you can use that information for future telephone calls, follow-up calls, and your marketing program.

10. **Take messages properly.** All messages must be complete and legible. Make sure you take down the full name and number of the caller. You don't want another staff person hunting around for the correct number or worse yet, making the call and using the wrong name of the original caller.

These 10 suggestions will help you provide better telephone service. Train your employees and yourself to develop a high skill level in all these areas. Your members will appreciate your service.

How to Say What You Say Even Better

Throughout my years as a consultant and trainer, I've heard people say some strange things on the telephone. Sometimes, the wording has been weird. Most of the time, however, it has to do with how the people are saying what they're saying. Based on the words and the tone being used, innocent comments, questions, and remarks can come off as very negative or sarcastic to members/customers.

I'm going to give you some examples of what people say on the phone and how to say the same things in better ways, but I need your help. Picture in your mind and listen in your head for different ways the following words can be said. More often than not, the tone of the voice messes up the entire mood of the conversation. One more thing, as you read the following situations, think about how it feels if you're on the receiving end of the remarks and how your customers feel when your staff talks in this manner.

> **How you say something conveys more meaning than what you say.**

Have you ever called up a club and asked to speak to a specific person and the receptionist or whomever answered the phone says, "Who's calling?" That's it. Nothing else. Just "Who's calling?" How does it make you feel? Do you feel uncomfortable? Out of sync? Strange? Think about how your members feel if this is done to them. A simple solution is to have your people ask "May I ask who's calling, please?" Or "May I have your name, please?" These comments soften the inquisition atmosphere. Similarly, when you hear "What is this in regard to?", you feel as though you're on the witness stand. Train your people to ask, "What is this in reference to, please?" or "May I please tell (the person's name) what this is in reference to?"

Here's one that I really love. You ask to speak to someone, and the receptionist tells you that person is not there. Then, she volunteers information that she doesn't know where the person is or when the person will be back. Some people even tell you that the person you want to speak to is in the bathroom. All they really have to say is "He/she is not in the office (in a meeting) and I expect him/her back at (a certain time)."

There are times when you have to leave your name and number for a return phone call. Instead of politely asking you, "May I have the correct spelling of your name and your phone number, please?" the person says, "What's your name and number?" How about when you're asking for information and the person says, "Lemme get that for you"? There are a number of better ways to say this: "Please hold while I get (obtain) that information for you." "Would

15 Telephone Tips and Reminders

1. Answer the phone by the third ring.

2. Greet the caller in a pleasant tone of voice by using your scripted greeting. Remember to include your name, your company's name, and your department.

3. When you get the caller's name, use it frequently in the conversation.

4. Listen carefully to get all the information the caller is providing. Take notes to ensure you don't forget anything.

5. Take the time to be helpful. When you cannot personally help the caller, ask their permission to put them on hold while you transfer the person to someone who will help.

6. Bridge the transfer of the call by telling the next staff person the caller's situation. Callers appreciate not having to be transferred around or having to repeat their stories.

7. Stress what you can do for callers. If, for any reason, you must refuse a request, explain why you cannot do what the caller asks at this time.

8. Say *please, thank-you,* and *you're welcome* during your conversations.

9. Return all calls promptly.

10. When you make a promise to a caller, keep it.

11. When you take a message for someone, get the caller's first and last name (have the caller spell them if necessary), the reason for the call, and the caller's phone number(s).

12. Never leave a caller on hold for more than 30 to 60 seconds without coming back on the line.

13. Treat all incoming calls as important ones. They could represent future business.

14. Always ask "Is there anything else I can do for you?" before you say good-bye.

15. Be proactive in your use of the phone. Use it to provide information to members, to gather feedback from members, and, of course, to sell memberships.

From Members for Life by Richard Gerson, 1999, Champaign, IL: Human Kinetics, copyright 1999 by Richard Gerson.

you mind holding while I get that for you?" "Please be patient while I get that information for you." Although these are all variations on the same theme, they do make a much better impression on the caller.

You call a club, or any business, and you're inquiring about a bill, for example. You state your case, and the staff person says something like "Yeah, our accounting department has been having a lot of screw ups lately." Or they say, "I don't know what to tell you about your bill. Accounting has been messing up a lot lately." Staff people should never make comments that put down another department in your club. What about when you call back for the second, third, or fourth time because a staff person never returned your call? The person who answers the phone says that the person whose call you were expecting never returns calls on time. Again, staff people should never put down another staff person to a caller. It gives a terrible impression of the club.

The last thing that shouldn't be said on the phone are words such as *yeah, uh-huh, nope*, and *un-un* (for no). Use *yes, no, I see, I understand*, or *I hear you* in place of slang phrases or grunts. Remember that you're a professional, and your staff members must represent your club in a professional manner. What they say on the phone and how they say it will definitely affect customers' perceptions of your club.

I know for myself that there are many times I've chosen not to do business with a company just because of the way I've been treated on the phone. There are many other times I've decided to buy from a company just because of the way they handled my telephone call. The telephone skills possessed by you and your employees can probably save many members who want to cancel their memberships or are just letting them lapse. A friendly and sincere voice on the phone does wonders.

The ultimate compliment related to telephone member service is when a member calls you up personally to tell you how wonderfully he was treated on the phone by one of your employees. When this happens, make sure you thank the member for taking the time to call, and then go right out and recognize the employee in a positive way. Make a big deal about this, because the reinforcement will motivate the employee to continue to provide great member service on the phone and in the club.

CHAPTER 6

The Service Recovery Process: Managing Angry Members and Complaining Members

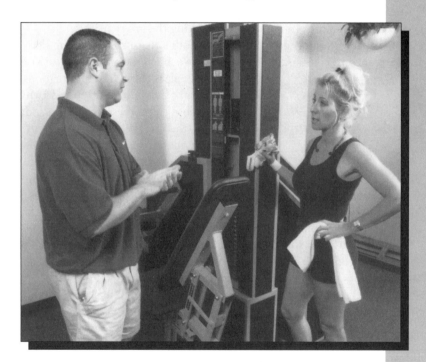

I n my role as a consultant, I get to do a lot of interesting and fun things. One client asked me to pretend I was an angry member. I had just joined the day before and came in earlier to work out, but I was told I couldn't work out because I didn't have a membership card and my name was not in the computer. These problems are easily resolved, but my client wanted to see how the front desk staff would react. I got very angry when I was told I couldn't work out, and I threatened to get them all fired. I even said I would file a lawsuit. One of the receptionists just turned away from me and ignored me while the other one continued to try to calm me down. Eventually, she succeeded, and I was quiet long enough to hear that I'd be allowed to work out that day without any problems.

We all have encountered angry members. Each member's anger is due to something different, but they are all angry just the same. How you handle them goes a long way to how well your club will be perceived by the members. A member could be angry for any number of reasons; I'll describe some of the most common ones later in the chapter. For now, think back to situations in your club where members were angry when they approached your staff. First, think about a situation where your staff did a great job of finding out why the member was angry and working to resolve the issues. Then consider a situation where your staff did a poor job of handling the angry member.

What things jump out at you from both situations? What similarities are there and what differences existed between the performances of your staff people in these difficult situations? Who asked the right questions, and what were those right questions? Who added fuel to the fire? Who in your club is the best at managing angry and complaining members, and what can you do to dupli-

A key to helping an angry member is listening.

cate those behaviors? The answers to these questions are important for every club owner and manager. This chapter will describe what makes members angry and what you can do about it. You'll also learn how to work with a complaining member and possibly even turn that situation into a sale.

Every club has its share of upset or angry members. I'm not talking about "the member from hell;" every club has its share of that type of person also. I'm talking about members who get angry over something that happened to them while in the club or related to the club's business. Some clubs deal with them well; others don't do well at all.

The surprising fact is that it's really very easy to manage angry members. The key is knowing exactly how to do it. Plus, you must know what they need from you right at the moment they are angry and what they expect of you after that. Before I get into the skills of handling upset members, let me give you a few other real-world examples from the fitness industry of how to effectively deal with an angry member, as well as how to totally blow the situation. The negative examples come first.

I was in a club several years ago, and a member was very upset about what she thought was an overcharge on her purchase in the pro shop. Now you and I both know that the bar code number is coded into the computerized cash register, and the price is rung up automatically. I'm sure the member knew this too. It didn't matter. This member was so sure she was overcharged on her purchase that she accused the cashier of cheating her. The poor cashier began to get flustered as she kept telling the shopper that the cash register rang up the cost automatically based on the coding. She had nothing to do with the prices. The member didn't care. She just kept yelling louder and louder that she was being cheated. As the volume level rose and the cashier started to cry, the pro shop manager came over (finally) to see what was going on.

You could tell the pro shop manager had no clue how to deal with an angry member. The member started yelling at the manager about being cheated. Instead of trying to calm her down and do something about the pricing for her, the manager yelled back, "If you don't like our prices, then don't shop here. We don't need your business anyway." What would you have done?

The next example involves a new club that opened up in the middle of a highly competitive area. Their membership prices were in line with the other clubs, although the new club was priced slightly higher. As prospective members came in to tour the club and join, they were presented with the membership prices. When they said that they could get the same or a better membership deal down the road, they received a great deal of pressure to join. As the prospective members became angry at the salespeople and complained to the owners about the high-pressure sales tactics, the new club owners told them, "Why don't you go to those other clubs? We're not changing our prices for anyone. We'll succeed without you being a member here." What would you have done?

Check out any club in any area of the fitness, country club, or hospitality industry when a member comes in to buy something and does not see what he or she wants or comes in with a complaint. In many cases, the person they're interacting with can't seem to deal with this member or provide the member with what he or she wants. Now the member begins to get irate, starts to yell, and gets angrier by the minute. The staff member either walks away, ignores the member, or yells back at the member.

Has this ever happened in your club? None of these examples are hard to believe. They happen all the time. Members receive less than appropriate treatment, and then they get angry. Or they feel they've been wronged in some way, and they get angry. Then when they try to take care of the situation, they don't receive any satisfactory resolution for their anger. That may be surprising to some of you because it has often been said that the member/customer is always right. (Here's something for you to consider: The member is not always right. For example, members who become verbally or physically abusive are definitely not right. The member is always the member, however.) The key question is what will you and your employees do to handle the angry member?

> *The entire service recovery process is based on effective communication.*

The first thing you must realize is that angry members want to be listened to and understood more than anything else. Listening to them shows that you respect them as people and are treating them in a dignified manner. Although this may sound too psychological or too philosophical, it's exactly what they want from you.

I had a client who asked me to arrange and promote his grand opening party for his club. We agreed in writing to a fee, plus all related expenses. When I presented him with the invoice, he started to get upset that he had to reimburse me $45 for expenses. He said that he was paying for my services, and he shouldn't have to pay for related expenses, even though he signed an agreement. I listened to him and calmly reminded him that he agreed to reimburse me for expenses, but that got me nowhere. He continued to get upset, so I asked him what must I do to make him feel better and to satisfy his concern over paying the expenses. He said that if I wiped the $45 off the invoice, he'd be very happy. So I did.

Now, $45 was not a lot of money to either of us. Principle was involved here, as well as the provision of great customer service. Just by asking him what I could do for him, listening to his answer, and then taking action on his answer, I calmed him down and kept a satisfied client. Would you have done the same thing I did? Would you have done anything different or additional?

This final example shows you that I'm human when I'm a customer too. This one comes from another industry, so you'll have to make the leap to apply it to your club. My wife took our children to a popular fast-food restaurant for dinner while I was on a business trip. When I returned the next day, she told me that they had to wait 20 minutes to get their order and that there were three things wrong with the order when they finally got it. When the restaurant tried to correct the problem, there was still something wrong with the meal, so they spent a total of 45 minutes in the restaurant to finish their meal. Plus, when my wife complained to the manager on duty, she received a very short and obnoxious response as if it were her fault that the problems occurred.

I got upset because we do visit that restaurant quite often. (It's the kids, you know.) I called up the restaurant and spoke with someone who was absolutely no help. I told him that I wanted to meet with the general manager. He told me when the manager would be in, and I said I would be there. When I met with the general manager, she did everything perfectly to handle me as an irate customer. She listened to me, apologized for what happened, and then calmly asked me what would make me happy. I told her that my family expects prompt and courteous service and treatment and that the meals should come out right the first time. She agreed and asked that we give the restaurant another chance by coming in for dinner anytime we wanted, for free. What would you have done?

These examples show you the good and the bad sides of dealing with angry members/customers. In a nutshell, you should listen carefully, calm members down, and find out what you must do to satisfy them. After you give them what they want, offer them something extra and unexpected to motivate them further to continue to do business with you. The following sections will help you get a better understanding of what angry members are thinking and feeling. You'll find out what they could be upset about (and it may have nothing to do with you, your club, or what they bought from you) and what they want from you when they are upset. You'll also learn a 10-step process to follow to help you better manage your angry members.

Why Members May Be Upset

Members could be upset for a variety of reasons. Some of the reasons have to do with their memberships; other reasons are more personal. You can find out what is bothering members by noticing their appearance and physical posture when they approach you and then asking appropriate questions. A comprehensive list of why members can be upset appears on the next page. Take a look at your club and see which of these items apply and whether there are any other reasons you need to add to the list. Make your employees aware of these potentially volatile situations and train them how to handle them.

What Members Want From You When They Are Angry

Knowing what is upsetting your members is very important. It is just as important to know what they want from you when they are angry. You already know that if they're upset and complaining about something that they want their complaint resolved. Every situation is unique, and you must handle it as such.

In the section on managing complaints, I talk about the five-step process of service recovery: apologize, restate the problem, empathize, make restitution, and follow up. This process also holds true whenever you encounter an angry member. You must always follow this five-step process. You must also understand that it's very important to give the angry members what they need psychologically and behaviorally in this situation.

On a personal level, members who are angry and complaining want certain things from you. They want to be

Listened to

Understood

Empathized with

Respected and have their dignity and integrity maintained

Valued

Made to feel important

Made to feel right

Made to feel intelligent

25 Reasons Members May Be Upset

1. They are in a hurry.

2. Their expectations have not been met.

3. They are already upset at someone else.

4. They are tired, stressed out, or frustrated.

5. They feel helpless, powerless, or victimized.

6. They feel no one listens to them.

7. They have a need to prove they're always right.

8. They have a chip on their shoulder for one reason or another.

9. They are promised something that is not delivered.

10. They are treated poorly or discourteously.

11. They are told to do two different things by two separate staff members.

12. They are told to do something by a staff member and it is wrong.

13. They feel someone in the club has a poor attitude toward them.

14. No one pays attention to them.

15. They have personal prejudices toward you or your staff.

16. They want to control or manipulate you by making a lot of noise.

17. They don't trust anyone in the club, or they have their integrity questioned by a staff member.

18. They are told not to be angry, which only makes them angrier.

19. They are spoken to in a disrespectful manner.

20. Your staff member argues with them.

21. They are confused, overwhelmed, nervous, anxious, or worried.

22. Their ego or self-esteem has been deflated.

23. They feel everyone in life treats them poorly, and they're taking it out on you.

24. They have to wait too long for something.

25. They are angry for no good or apparent reason.

Appreciated by their club

Taken seriously

Assured the problem will not happen again

Guaranteed immediate action

Relieved of their anger and anxiety

Compensated in some way

Remember what it's like when you're a member and you get angry. How are you treated? How does that make you feel? What did you want that service provider to do differently? What would you have done differently if you were the service provider instead of the member?

What to Do When the Member Is Angry

Here is the 10-step process I mentioned that you should follow whenever you encounter an angry member. Remember that managing the angry member also includes the service recovery process in some form. You'll see how it comes into play here, and I'll describe it in more detail later.

1. **Don't argue.** Acknowledge the member's right to be angry and upset.

2. **Listen carefully.** Allow the member to speak and completely ventilate his or her feelings. Although it may seem like an eternity, give the member anywhere from 30 seconds to two minutes of uninterrupted talk time. You'll find that most people can't sustain a high level of emotional anger for this long if you're just listening without interrupting. Use your active, reflective, and empathic listening skills to encourage the person to keep talking.

3. **Apologize and use reflective communication skills.** Tell the member you're sorry and restate the problem as you understand it. Also, let angry members know that you're going to do everything possible to help them because you want them to get over their anger.

4. **Show empathy.** Let angry members know you understand the problem from their point of view and sympathize with how they're feeling.

5. **Ask questions.** You must ask questions to get clarification on the problem and the member's interpretation of it. You have to make certain that you completely understand the situation, from the member's perspective as well as yours. Asking questions keeps you from making a statement that the member may perceive as placing the blame elsewhere or passing along the responsibility to resolve the issue.

6. **Thank the member.** That's right, say thank-you to the member for bringing the issue to your attention. Remember that only a small portion of your members take the time to complain, so you should treat every complaint or "angry encounter" as an improvement opportunity. When someone helps you get better, you thank that person.

7. **Make restitution.** Explain exactly what you're going to do to resolve the issue. Do this only after you've calmed the member down and he or she is now speaking with you rather than yelling or venting at you. After you explain what you're going to do, make sure the member understands what will be done and be certain the member is willing to accept your efforts.

8. **Do what you promise.** You must deliver on your promise of restitution. This situation is another opportunity to cement a member's loyalty. If you underpromise and overdeliver, the member will love you for life. If you don't do what you promised, you will never get another chance.

9. **Follow up.** Follow-up is essential to your continued success. Angry members may be feeling better for the moment when they leave you, but it's up to you to make certain their angry feelings don't resurface and return later. Call them or write them to make certain they still feel good about what you did for them.

10. **Give them something.** It can be a discount on their next purchase, something for free, or anything you can think of. The important thing is that members believe you've gone out of your way for them when they were angry and that you really want them to be satisfied and loyal members because you're willing to give them a gift to thank them for staying with you.

There's your 10-step process for dealing with and diffusing (and de-fusing) an angry member.

The entire service recovery process is based on effective communication. Use the following few service-related phrases to help you even more: (These phrases work well in any interpersonal situation where a disagreement has occurred.)

"I agree with you that . . ."

"I appreciate that . . ." or "I appreciate your . . ."

"I respect that . . ." or "I respect you for . . ."

"I understand . . ."

"You're right."

Using these agreement or bridge phrases will improve all aspects of your communication.

WHAT TO DO WHEN THE MEMBER IS ANGRY

1. Don't argue.
2. Listen carefully.
3. Apologize and use reflective communication skills.
4. Show empathy.
5. Ask questions.
6. Thank the member.
7. Make restitution.
8. Do what you promise.
9. Follow up.
10. Give them something.

Turning Complaints Into Sales

For many years, businesses, including health clubs, believed that customer service was nothing more than handling complaints. That's why many businesses had their customer service department (read complaint department) locked in a back room or off somewhere so that a complaining customer would not disturb other people. It's only recently that businesses have realized the importance of proactive customer service and that complaint management is an integral part of their success.

The concept of complaint management is the process of service recovery and restitution. Basically, you do whatever it takes to resolve the member's problem and make him or her happy. You also do it promptly, because the faster you resolve a member's complaint, the greater the likelihood that member will maintain his or her membership and stay loyal to you. What people and companies forget to do with their complaint management process is to use it as both a proactive service tool and a sales tool. You can turn a complaint situation into a sales situation; I give you a list of tactics to do so later in this chapter. First, I want you to read about some missed opportunities. These are all true stories.

I was a member of a club, and I brought two friends in for a tour. I mentioned to the front desk that these were prospective members and they wanted to see a sales counselor. Because no one was available, I conducted the tour and then returned to the front desk. There was still no sales counselor available, so my

Seven Types of Difficult Members and How to Manage Them Effectively

You are going to run into all types of members in your club, not just angry ones. It's true that the angry ones are the members you'll remember the most and the ones who'll probably give you the most trouble. However, there are also six other types of difficult members I've identified for you to consider. Your goal in dealing with each of these types is to make sure the member comes away feeling positive about you and your club. Keep in mind what I said before. The member may not always be right, but the member is always the member. Your job in dealing with all these different types of members and managing them, especially the angry ones, is to resolve their problems quickly and to their satisfaction. The result will be increased member loyalty and retention.

MEMBER TYPE	ACTION
The Angry Member	Listen.
	Don't argue.
	Avoid letting your emotions or the situation get to you.
	Show respect and treat the member with dignity.
	Ask tactful questions to identify the root of the problem.
	Offer positive, constructive solutions.
The Impatient Member	Respond quickly to requests.
	Get down to business immediately. Omit details unless the member requests them.
	Reassure the member that you will take care of the situation completely and on time, and that the job will be done right the first time.
	Make the member feel important. (Do this for all members all the time.)
The Confused Member	Find out exactly what is causing the confusion.
	Use sincerity to gain trust.
	Keep explanations brief and to the point. Focus on one item at a time to prevent further confusion.

	Reassure the member about the proper decision.
	Be patient and provide guidance and further reassurance.
The Frightened Member	Do whatever you can and must to alleviate the fear, once you know exactly what it is and what's causing it.
	Speak calmly and softly.
	Build trust with your sincere offers to help.
	Offer simple explanations.
	Reassure the member that everything will be fine and that you'll stay with him or her until the fear subsides.
The Insulted Member	Apologize.
	Be calm and brief.
	Reassure the member in a positive manner.
	Listen as the member talks out the situation.
	Follow up with full explanations as to your actions and resolutions.
The Interrupting Member	Ask not to be interrupted.
	Be firm, be brief, and be polite.
	Give explanations of key points.
	Maintain your conversational tone of voice.
	Show restraint and model appropriate communications behaviors.
The Talkative Member	Listen.
	Be polite, yet firm.
	Apologize and explain your time constraints and your reasons for leaving the conversation.
	Focus on giving the member what he or she wants.
	Tell the member you'll get back to him or her in a specific number of minutes with a response.

Now you know how to identify and manage angry members, as well as deal with other types of difficult members. Handle these people with care. The outcome of your tender handling can result in these members being so satisfied with how you treated them that they stay with you for life. The success of your club is in your hands when it comes to managing these types of members. Do whatever is necessary, and train your staff to do the same.

friends were asked to wait for a few minutes. Those few minutes turned into 30 minutes, so my friends just walked out.

The front desk never tried to stop them, nor did anyone from membership sales ever ask me who they were. Obviously, this club had no clue about the concept of service recovery and restitution. You can be sure my friends never came back. Contrast this with a similar situation in another club (different city, different year) where the manager came out, apologized for the delay, offered two weeks' worth of free guest passes, and invited my friends to come back another time. This manager turned a poor service situation into an additional sales opportunity through his recovery efforts.

Here's another story: A club had not refurbished its locker room area for many years, and members were complaining about the appearance and the odor. The club's management either didn't want to hear about the problems, or they just hoped the problems would go away. Nothing was done regarding the complaints. After several months, one of the members threatened legal action against the club, saying it was not delivering on its promises of a safe and healthy environment for its members. Still, the club did not respond. Although no legal action was taken, this member and dozens of others let their memberships lapse and joined elsewhere. It seems to me that the club ran its business for its own convenience rather than that of the member. Do you run your club that way? Or do you do whatever it takes to effectively manage complaints and turn them into sales?

Here is a simple, step-by-step process to effectively manage complaints and create satisfied customers. Following that, I'll provide you with the method for turning complaints into sales. Always remember that customers whose complaints are resolved quickly and to their satisfaction are the most motivated buyers you will ever run into. They may not buy from you immediately, but the odds are in your favor that they will eventually buy from you. Be proactive in handling all your customer complaints, go through the recovery and restitution process, and turn the complaints into sales.

Service recovery and restitution is usually a five-step process. Members who complain or who are dissatisfied either feel annoyed, cheated, or victimized. They also feel that their situation is the most important in the world. You must be aware of this attitude and treat them accordingly. Remember that dissatisfied members tell up to 20 friends that they are unhappy with the way you do business and run your club. However, if you resolve their problems, between 50 and 80 percent of these same members will renew their memberships with you.

Club Service Recovery and Restitution Program

Adapt the following five-step recovery program to your club and specific situation. Also, remember to train your employees on this process.

1. **Apologize.** First and foremost, apologize for the inconvenience the member has experienced. Be sincere and genuine with the apology. The member will notice if you are just going through motions to make this apology. Also, a sincere apology usually tends to defuse any additional anger the member may have.

2. **Restate the problem.** To make certain you understand exactly what the member means, restate the problem as the member described it to you. Then tell the member and show the member, if possible, that you will do everything possible to solve the problem and re-solve the complaint. Even if you are unable to resolve the problem to the member's full-est satisfaction, the member will perceive that you were sincere

> *Customers whose complaints are resolved quickly and to their satisfaction are the most motivated buyers.*

and definitely intended to help. The member's dissatisfaction may not disappear, but his or her level of being dissatisfied will certainly diminish.

3. **Empathize.** Make certain you communicate clearly to members so that they understand that you understand how they feel. Do not patronize or try to pacify them. Just show them and tell them that you understand how they feel. Make sure you express yourself well so that the member does not confuse empathy with sympathy or pity.

4. **Make restitution.** Here is your chance to make points. Not only are you going to take immediate action to resolve the complaint, such as giving the member's money back, extending his or her membership, or making an exchange or offering a credit in your pro shop, you are going to go a step further. Tell and show the member you will make it up to him or her in some special way. Give the member a gift, or let the member purchase a new item at a sale price (additional member-ship time, for example). Whatever you do, look at it as adding value and keeping a loyal member rather than spending extra money.

5. **Follow up.** This step is where most programs fail. You or your staff neglect to follow up with the member to ensure that member is satisfied. It can be a simple question or two asked at the end of the recovery process: "Have I resolved your complaint to your satisfaction? What else can I do for you?" Then wait a few days and call the member on the telephone to make certain he or she is still satisfied. You can also send the member a letter. A nice touch would be to enclose a coupon or gift certificate with the letter. Again, going the extra mile will help you create and keep a loyal member.

This is the basic five-step approach to service recovery and restitution. You may want to break the restitution step down into resolution (the action taken to resolve the complaint) and restitution (anything else that you do for the member to make up for the problem). Whatever you do, use this approach as a guide and develop a workable program for your club. This approach also helps you to consider service recovery and restitution as more than just part of a complaint management program. Recovery and restitution can become one of your many tactics for long-term member retention.

Managing Complaints for Member Retention

You now know the basics for handling a complaint and keeping a member. You should also look at this situation as a unique sales opportunity. Members are more motivated to buy from you right at the time you have taken special care of them (resolved their complaint) than at any other time. Once you have resolved the complaint to their satisfaction, you can begin working on a new sale. Remember that when you do this, you are creating a loyal and long-term member. Here are 10 suggestions on how to turn member complaints into additional sales:

1. Understand why the member is complaining. Someone, somehow has not met the member's expectations for something or satisfied a particular need.

2. Listen attentively to the entire complaint without interrupting the member. Providing undivided attention during this monologue shows the member that you respect him or her.

3. Handle one complaint at a time even if the member has several complaints. You will manage one complaint more effectively if you concentrate on it alone instead of trying to do too many things at once.

4. Ask the member what's different about his or her situation now. Have previous needs changed? When you know the discrepancy, you can take steps to resolve it.

5. Apologize and demonstrate empathy. Then assure the member you will do everything possible to resolve the issue.

6. Always discuss new sales opportunities and benefits as soon as you resolve the initial complaint.

7. Treat a complaint situation as a sales situation. Probe, provide information, handle objections, and close.

8. Close confidently. Just because this sale is coming from the resolution of a complaint, you cannot be apologetic in your close. You are still offering benefits that will help the member.

9. If you cannot resolve the complaint to the member's satisfaction, turn the member over to someone else. If no one can resolve the complaint, ask the member what you should do.

10. Know that over three-fourths of your complaining members will stay with you if you resolve their complaints quickly. Use this knowledge to your benefit and consider their complaints as free consulting.

These 10 suggestions will help you manage complaints and turn them into additional sales. Perhaps even more importantly, you will show members that you care about them. Remember that they don't care how much you know until they know how much you care. Combine your complaint management process with the service recovery and restitution process, and you will increase your sales, increase member satisfaction, and keep your members for life.

CHAPTER 7

Three Critical Customer Service Skills: Building Rapport, Interpersonal Communication, and Effective Listening

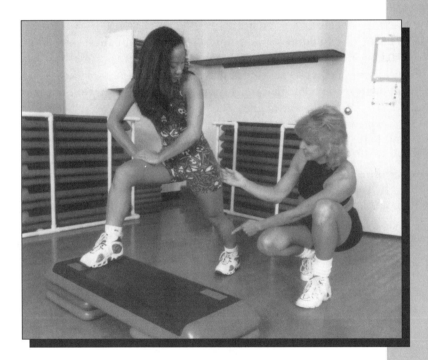

N ow that we've looked at using the telephone effectively in your club, handling angry members, and managing complaints, it's time to focus on the foundation skills that help you perform those functions. Whenever you interact with a member, you need to establish rapport, communicate clearly and effectively, and listen to what the member is saying and not saying.

Think about the last time you were speaking with someone, but things just didn't seem right. Either or both of you were uncomfortable. It seemed the whole scene was taking place somewhere else. Neither of you was really listening carefully to the other, and you both couldn't wait to get the conversation over with. What was the problem? Put simply, you were out of rapport. You were not communicating on the same wavelength, and this miscommunication made it difficult for you to listen to each other.

Now, think about how members feel when they're trying to communicate with you and the two of you are out of touch. The member may want to tell you something positive about the club, or something negative, or just ask for information. You may be preoccupied, or have a previous opinion about this member, or not have the time to be bothered right now. Whatever the case is, the words you and the member use and the body language you both exhibit will make it difficult to communicate.

That's why building rapport, interpersonal communication, and effective listening are three of the most important skills you can possess to provide great customer/member service and to make members want to stay with you for life. I strongly recommend that you do not offer training in only one or two of these skills to the exclusion of the others. Success in customer service and the subsequent effects on member retention are based on a systems approach to skill building. This type of approach means that an interactive effect exists among all the skills and that they all are taught and practiced for effective performance.

Many people will say that building rapport, communication, and listening are all part of the same skill set. I would agree, to a point. Although these skills can all come under the heading of communication, they are distinct skills that must be addressed separately. I can tell you that my clients have achieved greater performance improvements and received much better results when I've trained their employees by separating the three skills instead of lumping them together. I know this because the members at these clubs give higher satisfaction ratings. Let's take a look at each skill individually.

Building Rapport

Building rapport is essential for a successful customer interaction with your members. Rapport leads to credibility and trust, friendliness, and a feeling of comfort. As an exercise, think back to a situation where you were with someone who made you feel uncomfortable. Your body became tense, you didn't think as clearly as you normally would, and you just knew things weren't right. Your greatest hope was to find a way out of the situation. Conversely, think of someone with whom you get along very well. You're very comfortable together. It's as if you both know what the other is going to say before it's said.

You seem to know what each person is thinking or feeling. You just click. The reason for all these positive feelings and perceptions is that you're in rapport.

Because we all want to feel good, and as fitness professionals, we pride ourselves on helping other people feel good, we should always try to be in rapport with our members. How do we develop this rapport, and how do we do it rapidly in a member service situation?

Follow this sequence of actions and you'll find yourself able to develop rapport with members, and everyone else, almost instantly. As the member approaches you (or you approach the member), notice everything you can about that person: appearance, clothes, cologne or perfume, hair color, and jewelry. Greet the member with a smile and an enthusiastic hello. You should have already learned the member's name, and you must use it several times at the beginning of your conversation. Say something nice about the member, especially regarding her appearance (or

> **Greet members with a smile and an enthusiastic hello.**

anything else). Pay attention to the posture and body language of the member and begin to mirror that: Stand as she does or fold your arms as she does. Just make sure your body language and posture is similar to hers. When the member speaks, notice the rate and pitch of the speech. When it's your turn to talk, mirror her speech patterns as closely as possible without mimicking them. When the member speaks, you listen attentively.

Review this sequence in order:

1. The member approaches, and you notice everything you can about the member.

2. You greet the member with a smile and an enthusiastic hello.

3. You use the member's name several times during the initial parts of the conversation.

4. You notice his body language and mirror it.

5. You notice his rate of speech and modify yours accordingly.

6. You match the pitch and tone of his voice, using as many similar words as possible.

7. You listen carefully and attentively to what the member is saying.

Although this may seem like a lot for you to do, consider how long it will take for you to do this. The answer is not long at all. The first 15 to 30 seconds of every member encounter is all the time you need to establish rapport. If you follow the previous seven steps, you should get into rapport in no time at all. When these skills become a habit for you, they will occur naturally. You won't even be aware of any energy being expended on your part to build rapport with your members. You'll even get so good at building rapport that you'll be able to do it with several people at once. The members will love you for it, even if they can't explain it. Plus, it will help you move through all your communication interactions with the members.

Interpersonal Communication

There are hundreds of books that tell you how to communicate more effectively. Without trying to write the next one, this section will identify for you some of the most important interpersonal communication skills you must develop in order to provide superior member service. Remember that you can use these skills in all aspects of your service encounters, as well as to improve your relationships with other people.

The first thing you must decide on is your communication stance with regard to members. Are you going to take the "resist stance" or the "assist stance"? Although the choice should seem obvious, you can't deny the fact that some employees in clubs still believe they could do a great job if only the members wouldn't get in the way. Some people just want to be contrary or create conflict; others can't wait to help and be of service. Which one are you? Which approach fits your employees? Without trying to influence you, I recommend you take the assist stance.

Once you do this, you must be aware that effective communication is only defined by the response you receive. Effective communication has nothing to do with what you are saying, although that is important. Suppose you ask a member to go to register A to pay for a purchase. That instruction seems pretty straightforward and easy to understand. But the member goes to register B instead. The member obviously did not follow your directions, and the member may not have understood your instructions. As hard as this may be to believe, it is true. Just because what you say seems clear to you, it may not be clear to a member or any other person you're communicating with.

This next example clearly illustrates the differences people have in interpreting the meaning of a communication. Suppose you and I are talking, and it's Tuesday morning. We decide to meet for lunch next Wednesday. I put it in my calendar for eight days away, because next Wednesday to me means the following week. You, on the other hand, perceive it to mean the next Wednesday coming up (tomorrow in this example). We don't check on our interpretations of "next Wednesday," and you show up at the appointed time and place tomorrow. I'm not there; you're upset that I stood you up; and we may have an argument about who was right or wrong.

Extend this scenario to you and a member. The member wants to meet with you "next Wednesday" to discuss some changes in his or her membership program. Because it is Tuesday morning, you simply assume that you'll meet in eight days. Neither of you confirms the interpretation of "next Wednesday."

The member shows up tomorrow at the appointed time. You're either not there or busy with someone else. The member is upset and doesn't understand how you could misinterpret the day and time of the appointment. In reality, you didn't. You misinterpreted (in the member's mind) the date of the appointment.

These two brief examples show you how important it is to clarify the intent of your message as it relates to the response you are getting from the member. Even if the member correctly interpreted what you said, his or her behavior in response to your instructions made your communication ineffective. That's why it's imperative for you as an effective communicator to simultaneously be aware of the effect you want from your communication and the response you actually receive.

If you are the one speaking or writing, and you don't get the desired effect, you, not the member or employee who is the recipient of your communication, need to change your words, your behavior, or your approach. Don't keep trying to communicate in the same way if it is obviously not working. Remember the definition of insanity: Doing the same thing over and over again in the same way and expecting different results. You as the service provider should always adapt to the member rather than the other way around. Applying these basic tips will help you communicate more effectively in all types of member service and other interpersonal situations.

10 Keys to Effective Communication

In teaching interpersonal communication skills in a variety of settings, I've found that there are 10 key elements to effective communication. When you learn these 10 keys and incorporate them into your communication repertoire, you will become more effective and persuasive as a communicator:

1. **Pay attention.** Give the speaker your undivided attention.

2. **Be adaptable and flexible.** Be ready and able to change what you're doing to improve communication.

3. **Make eye contact.** You've got to look at people when you communicate with them.

4. **Ask questions.** The only way you learn something is to ask about it. Remember that ask stands for "always seek knowledge."

5. **Listen.** No one ever learned anything by talking. Listen twice as much as you speak. After all, you have two ears and one mouth. Effective communicators use these sense organs in those proportions.

6. **Use stories, analogies, and metaphors.** People communicate more effectively and remember more of what was communicated by using these indirect methods rather than simply stating facts. People love hearing about or reading stories and examples, and they also like to

make the leap from analogies and metaphors to their own lives. Learn to use these communication devices, and you'll become a much more effective communicator. (Think about how many stories, analogies, and metaphors you've already read in this book.)

7. **Mirror and match the other person's speech and body language.** When you match another person's body language and speech patterns as closely as possible without mimicking them, that person perceives that you are very much like he or she is, and he or she starts to like and trust you immediately. You get into rapport almost instantly.

8. **Build rapport.** You've got to build trust as quickly as possible to open up all the lines of communication. Rapport is the key to building trust when communicating.

9. **Understand pacing and leading.** These two techniques are used to develop an effective communication. With pacing, you follow the other person's lead by matching his or her verbal and nonverbal behavior. When you're leading, the other person is matching whatever you are doing.

10. **Respond appropriately.** Know when to respond and what to say. Sometimes, your nonverbal responses say more than your verbal/vocal responses.

These 10 keys to effective communication will definitely help you work better with employees and members. Most of the people who succeed in life are effective and persuasive communicators. When you think about almost every member service encounter, or any other interpersonal interaction, the major component is communication between two or more people.

Effective Listening

You've already figured out that I'm a firm believer in communicating clearly, succinctly, and effectively with your members. Up to this point, I've talked about you being the initiator in the communication, but the most important skill you can develop, and the one your members will appreciate the most, is the ability to listen.

Because your goal is to serve and satisfy member needs, you've got to find out what those needs are. If you want to find out exactly what your members need, want, and expect from you, you can't presume to know what each individual needs. Lumping members into categories as you're providing service to them is not fair either. The key to finding out this important information is to ask them. When you ask them, listen carefully to their verbal responses and watch carefully for their nonverbal responses.

All too often, I've been involved with people in companies who ask questions and then don't wait for or listen to the answer. You probably know a few people like that, too. Doesn't it aggravate and annoy you when they ask you something and then don't even have the courtesy to allow you time to completely answer their questions? Or they ask the question of you and then answer it themselves. If it annoys you, how do you think your members feel if you or an employee do this to them?

Your members feel the same way as you do. It's vitally important that you listen to all your members. Everyone has something important to say to you, either personally or in writing. By listening to your members, you get some of the best free consulting advice anywhere. Their comments and feedback are quite often indications of what you can do to improve your club. That's what customer service is all about. Remember that service and selling are all about people and their relationships.

During a sales training seminar I conducted a while back, I had just completed a role play with one of the attendees. When we finished, this sales professional "insulted" me by saying I was more service-oriented than sales-oriented. She told me that I spent more time listening to her during the role play (I was the salesperson and she was the customer) than telling her about my product. She got the impression that I was more interested in establishing a business relationship with her company and providing them with great service than I was in pushing for a sale right then and there. She was right. I thanked her profusely because I'm a firm believer that your attitude toward building

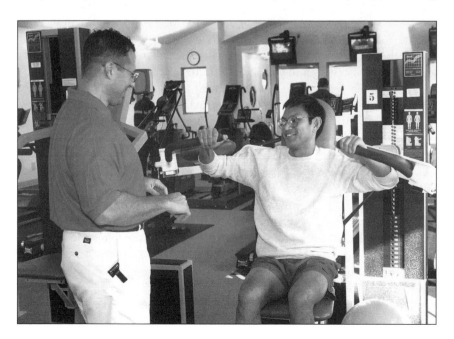

relationships and providing customer service will come across during your sale. People will be more likely to buy from you once, and then again, when you listen to them. It shows you care about them. In order to be customer service-oriented and retain members for life, you have to be an effective listener.

Listening Is a Skill

Listening is a skill that is learned. Hearing is what you are born with. Listening is what you do with your hearing. It involves your perception and interpretation of what you hear.

The first thing you must do as an effective listener is pay attention to the speaker. Focus on who the person is and what that person is saying. Give the person your undivided attention so you can clearly hear the message. Then, you must interpret the message in light of your own perceptions, experiences, and the context in which the message was sent. This interpretation allows you to evaluate the message and make a judgment on what it means to you. When you get to this point, you've listened. Next, you provide feedback to the speaker (or writer) by acknowledging you understand what he or she was trying to communicate and responding to the message.

There are four types of listening that you can do: active listening, passive listening, reflective listening, and empathic listening. *Active listening* is when you are physically and vocally involved with the speaker. You motivate them to continue speaking by saying things such as "Yes, I understand" or "Go on" or by simply nodding your head in agreement or even smiling at them as they speak. All these things are signs that you are paying attention and listening and you want them to continue.

Listen to your members.

In a customer service situation, you must listen actively. The last thing a member wants from you as the service provider is for you to be inattentive, have your attention wander, or act as though you're disinterested. The member should be the center of your world when he or she is there in front of you or on the phone with you. Nothing should distract you unless it's vitally important, and even then you must weigh the situation. Otherwise, pay attention to the member and be actively involved with whatever the member is speaking about.

If the member is asking you questions, the only way you can provide accurate answers is to listen carefully to the questions. Make sure you know what the member is asking, and that you interpret the words the same way the member means them. If the member is complaining about something, the only way you can resolve the complaint is to listen. If the member is just making conversation, the only way you can make the member feel comfortable is to establish rapport and listen.

When members are comfortable with you, they trust you more. When they trust you more, they like you more and buy more from you. When members are comfortable with a service provider, they will allow that person more leeway if some type of mistake is made. Because we're all human, we know that everyone makes mistakes from time to time. So be active and involved when you converse with members.

The type of listening you don't want to demonstrate in front of a member is called *passive listening*. With passive listening, you're still listening, but you're not showing any signs of life. You're just there. You hear everything that's being said. You take it in, evaluate it, and maybe formulate your response. You may even be thinking, "When is this going to end?" But whatever is going on inside of you, you don't give any indication that you're involved with what the member is saying. The member then starts to get turned off because he or she doesn't know where you're coming from or whether you're truly paying attention to him or her.

If passive listening is your preferred style, I suggest you change it immediately if you want to be able to provide superior member service and retain more members. Remember that a majority of people stop doing business with a company because they don't like the way the staff treated them. This bad treatment usually translates into staff members not listening to customers. Practice your active listening skills on family and friends and ask them for honest feedback. Work hard to improve this aspect of your behavior, and you'll find that your member satisfaction will improve.

After you develop your active listening skills and get rid of your passive listening skills, you move on to higher order listening skills. The first of these

10 Keys to Effective Communication

1. Pay attention.

2. Be adaptable and flexible.

3. Make eye contact.

4. Ask questions.

5. Listen.

6. Use stories, analogies, and metaphors.

7. Mirror and match the other person's speech and body language.

8. Build rapport.

9. Understand pacing and leading.

10. Respond appropriately.

is *reflective listening*. In reflective listening, you're actively listening to members and motivating them to continue their part of the conversation. When they take a break, you verbally reflect on what they've said by repeating it back to them or paraphrasing it. Or you simply say "Go on" or something of that nature to motivate the person to continue. This action on your part invites them to expand on that particular topic and to continue speaking. Reflective listening is a skill that many therapists, sales professionals, and consultants use to keep their clients talking. It also helps you deepen the rapport you've already established. You'd do well to develop this skill to improve your member service.

After you have reflective listening mastered, you can move on to what is called *empathic listening*. Empathic listening is when you communicate to the member that you truly understand their situation. You're displaying empathy (not pity or sympathy, empathy). Some phrases you might use to show empathy include "I understand" and "I know." Be careful what you say, however. For example, if you say "I know exactly how you feel," you'd better know exactly how that person feels. If you don't, that person will respond to you with something like, "How could you know exactly how I feel? Did this ever happen to you?" If it didn't, you can't know exactly how that person feels. Plus, you've just destroyed any trust you may have established.

> **Effective communication is only defined by the response you receive.**

Here's a real-world example. While I was working with a club, the management decided to let the marketing director go. This person had been with the club for four years, and the reason that was given was budget cuts. As the club's consultant, I happened to be working out of the marketing director's office. When she returned from being terminated, she was livid. I received the brunt of her anger even though I had nothing to do with it.

She proceeded to berate the club and even started yelling at me. She told me she and her husband just bought a new house and now they won't be able to pay for it. They're still trying to sell their old house, so they may be carrying two mortgages. I listened carefully, reflected on what she was saying, and then moved on to empathic listening by saying I understood how she felt. This statement only made her angrier, and she asked how I could understand how she felt. Was I going through the same thing she was? Now, she was even angrier because she thought I was pitying her.

I said I wasn't going through the same thing now, but that I had carried two mortgages for a while several years ago. Once I said that and she accepted it, her anger toward me dissipated, and we were able to discuss her situation more amicably. There was nothing I could do about her termination, but she knew I cared enough to listen. So although empathy is the highest order listening skill you can have, I hope this example shows you that you've got to temper it by being careful with your words.

In all the years I've done member service training and consulting, the one thing I've found to be consistent across people is their desire to be understood when they are speaking. Even if you disagree with what members are saying, show empathy first by letting them know you understand their feelings, where they're coming from, and what they are thinking before you begin to state your side of the situation. You can never persuade anyone over to your ideas unless you first acknowledge the validity of that person's position on a subject.

These, then, are the four types of listening that you can demonstrate: active, passive, reflective, and empathic. You want to get all the way to empathic listening with your members so they can develop a deeper feeling of rapport and trust with you. The more comfortable they feel around you, the more business they'll do with you. You need to pay attention to them and listen to them.

10 Things That Influence Your Listening to a Member

Go down the list of the following 10 things that can influence your listening to a member. Which ones can you control? Which ones can you control your reactions to? Which ones don't you care about or pay any attention to?

1. **Who the member is:** Is it a regular member? A big spender? A friend?
2. **The member's speaking style:** Is it fast or slow, to the point or dragged out?
3. **The member's appearance:** Well-dressed or shabby? Clean or dirty?
4. **Your past experiences with this member:** Good or bad? Friendly or unfriendly?
5. **Your mood:** Good or bad? Happy or sad? Friendly or unfriendly?
6. **Your health:** How do you feel? Are you taking care of yourself?
7. **The time and place of the conversation:** Your club? The member's home? Day or night?
8. **The setting or the situation:** Calm or tense? Inside or outside? Hot or cold?
9. **The perceived power of the member:** How does his or her purchase impact you?
10. **The importance to you of what the member is saying:** Is it meaningful for you?

These 10 things have a tremendous influence on your ability to listen to a member. Any one of them alone that becomes negative can cause you to miss something important that the member is saying. I know it seems like a lot of things to think about just to be an effective listener, but don't worry. As you develop your listening skills, these things begin to fall into place naturally.

Think back to a positive member service situation where you handled the situation to the member's total and complete satisfaction. When you were speaking to that member, didn't you do all of the following?

Refrain from interrupting the member?

Do everything possible to put the member at ease?

Concentrate on what the member was saying?

Remove all possible distractions while you listened?

Show empathy for the member's situation?

Pay attention to what was being said?

Pay attention to the nonverbal cues to find the real meaning of the member's message?

Control your emotions, especially if you disagreed with something the member said?

Refrain from making any judgments before you heard all the details?

Ask questions to get more information, to keep the member talking, and to help you better understand the member's situation?

Provide feedback to the member to show you understood exactly what was being said?

I know that there have been many member service situations, and other situations throughout your life, when your answer to all these questions would be a resounding yes. You've done it before without ever thinking about it. You can do it again, and do it constantly.

Go back to chapter 6, which explained how to handle angry or complaining members. One of the most important things they want from you is to be listened to without interruption. It's the same for someone who comes up to you and strikes up a conversation. They want to know that when they extend the courtesy of listening to you, you'll do the same for them. You should expect no less from someone you start talking with. You owe it to each other to listen.

In order to provide great member service, and keep members coming back, you need to be an effective listener. Many times, this can be the difference between a member staying with you or going to a competitor. If you do a new member survey for your club, and you probe deeply enough with your questions, you may find that many of your new members left their previous clubs because no one listened to them or paid attention to them. It's amazing how an everyday skill such as listening can mean the difference between a successful and an unsuccessful business.

CHAPTER 8

Measuring Member Satisfaction, Retention, and Loyalty

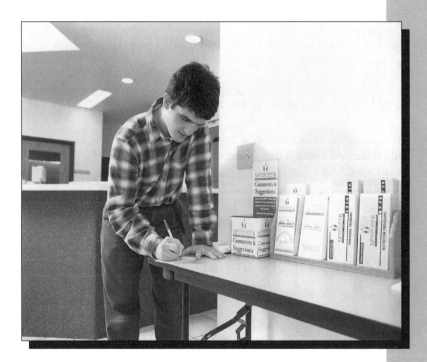

A great deal of information is being published and discussed on the topic of customer service, customer satisfaction, customer retention, and customer loyalty. Clubs and other businesses used to conduct surveys to find out whether their customers were satisfied. When they calculated their results, they'd find that x percent were extremely satisfied, and another percentage was somewhat satisfied. Based on their satisfaction ratings, they assumed they were doing a good job or needed improvements in some areas. What they didn't look at then, and are only starting to look at now, is that satisfied customers are not always loyal. They may take some of their business elsewhere.

But before you start worrying about the loyalty levels of your members, work on satisfying them first. Unless they are satisfied, they can't be retained, and they can't become loyal. The only thing that counts today, first, is customer satisfaction. If your customer is not satisfied, he or she will stop doing business with you.

Just what is customer satisfaction? It is the customer's perception that his or her expectations have been met or surpassed. You buy something, and you expect it to work properly. If it does, you are satisfied. If it does not, you are dissatisfied. If you are dissatisfied, it is up to the seller to find a way to fix the problem so that you can become satisfied. When the fix occurs to your approval, you are satisfied. When it does not, you will vote with your feet and take your business elsewhere.

Satisfied Customers Buy More and More Often

One simple truth of marketing is that satisfied customers do more business with you more often. They spend more on each purchase, and they purchase more often. They also refer their family and friends to you. The link between marketing, sales, service, satisfaction, and profits is direct. The more satisfied customers are, the more those customers spend. The more they spend, the more you sell. Usually, when you sell more, your profits are greater.

Which Is More Important: Quality, Service, Satisfaction, or Retention?

To ensure your success, your business must determine whether quality, service, satisfaction, or retention is most important. I will discuss how to measure all these aspects in a moment. For now, you must realize that they are all important, with certain distinctions. Quality and service are the means to the ends of satisfaction and retention. Your end goal in the club business should not be to produce a quality product or service or to provide superior customer service. These are just means to goals. Your ultimate goal should be to produce a satisfied and loyal customer who will stay with you (retention) over time. Therefore, providing high quality and superior customer service are givens when you consider what your ultimate goals are.

> *Satisfied customers buy more and more often.*

What Gets Measured Gets Done

Whenever you measure something, it gets performed, completed, and, usually, improved upon. That is why measurement techniques are so important to customer service and performance improvement. It is also why so many companies have begun measuring the satisfaction levels of their customers. When you have a quantifiable number or measure to put on a behavior, people can see exactly what effect that behavior is having on their own and the company's performance. Asking customers to rate you on your levels of quality and service and their level of satisfaction virtually guarantees that you will work to improve your efforts in these areas.

Defining Customer Satisfaction

The definition of customer satisfaction is very simple. A customer is satisfied whenever his or her needs, real or perceived, are met or exceeded. How do you know what the customer needs, wants, and expects? You ask! That's right. It's very simple. You just ask them, and then you give them what they want and more. Remember, when a product or service meets or exceeds a customer's expectations, the customer is usually satisfied.

Why We Measure Customer Satisfaction

Before you can measure something, you must know what you are measuring and why. The following material will introduce you to the reasons for measuring customer satisfaction. When you know why you are doing this, and then you do it, your implementation of the results of your measurement program will proceed more smoothly. Your measurement program must answer the who, what, when, where, how, and why questions that are essential for success:

Who will measure customer satisfaction? The answer is everyone.

What must be measured? Everything and anything that affects the customer/member.

When must you measure? All the time.

Where do you measure? Throughout the entire club and every process that has an effect on customer satisfaction and retention.

How do you measure? You establish performance standards and criteria that are quantifiable and that you can evaluate your performance against using hard numbers and data.

Why do you measure? You measure to learn how to improve performance and increase customer satisfaction.

There are seven basic reasons for conducting these measurements:

1. To learn about member perceptions
2. To determine customer needs, wants, requirements, and expectations
3. To close the gaps
4. To inspect what you expect in order to improve service and member satisfaction
5. Because improved performance leads to increased profits
6. To learn how you are doing and where you go from here
7. To apply the process of continuous improvement

The following sections explain these reasons in more detail.

Learning About Member Perceptions

Members are individuals, and each person will perceive things differently in the same situation. Although many measurement programs attempt to get at mass averages from which they will build or rebuild their customer service programs, you must also try to identify each customer's individual perceptions.

> *You can never know what a customer truly wants unless you ask.*

The perceptions you are trying to identify include what members look for in a club such as yours, why they would join your club, what has caused them to change clubs in the past, and what might make them change again in the future. You also try to discover their criteria for acceptable service quality, what they must receive from you to be minimally satisfied, what you must do to make them extremely satisfied, and what you must do for them so they will continue to do business with you.

Determining Customer Needs, Wants, Requirements, and Expectations

Your customer satisfaction measurements must not only determine how members feel about the product or service they purchased and the customer service they received, the measurement must also identify what the members need and want from you. You must also find out what they require of you in the way of program content, as well as what they expect you to provide during the overall sale and service experience.

It is vitally important to the success of your measurement program that you learn about members' current and future needs. Too many clubs that do these surveys ask about a recent purchase without ever trying to find out why members made the purchase, what personal and psychological need the purchase satisfied, how members plan to use the purchase, what members expect from the purchase, and what they expect their needs to be in the future.

Suppose you build mousetraps, and you have just built the best mousetrap the world has ever seen. Now someone once said that if you build a better mousetrap, the world (read customers) will beat a path to your door. That is assuming they need, want, and require a better mousetrap. If your customers have no need for mousetraps, now or in the future, they will not buy them from you. So now you have the world's greatest mousetrap and no customers. When you measure customer satisfaction, also measure what customers need, want, require, and expect from you and why.

Closing the Gaps

Many gaps exist between members' perceptions and the perceptions of you as the service provider. You must identify and measure gaps because this is the only way to close them. All the gaps are based on differences in perception between what the business believed has occurred and what the customer perceived to have received. Here is a list of several of the more important gaps that have been identified through research:

• **The gap between what a business thinks a customer wants and what the customer actually wants.** To understand this gap, just imagine that the company that built the better mousetrap decides it will inform the customers they need to buy it, but all the customer wants is a piece of cheese. You and your club can never know what a customer truly wants unless you directly ask the customer. Although your measurement tool may inform customers of what you think they may want, you must make it easy for them to tell you specifically what they want. The difference in perceptions is the gap you must close here.

• **The gap between what a business thinks a member has bought and what a member perceives has been received.** A line in a Broadway play said, "He sold him a horse, but he bought a mule." It really doesn't matter what the business sold to the customer if the customer perceives he or she did not receive exactly what was supposed to be purchased: a mule instead of a horse, a regular stereo instead of a surround-sound stereo, or a personal training program that promises one set of results but the member receives a different set of results. The gap exists because the customer does not perceive the purchase in the same way as the business perceives the purchase. Even if the business is right, the customer will feel cheated and be dissatisfied. (Have you had this situation occur in your club?) The business must close that gap and make certain the customer is satisfied.

- **The gap between the service quality the club believes it is providing and what the customer perceives is being provided.** This gap is very similar to the preceding gap in that the club believes one thing and the customer believes another. This gap usually occurs when the club has certain customer service policies that it tends not to change for each individual customer and neglects to inform the member of the policies. Thus, both parties are making decisions without benefit of all the available information. The customer does not know the club has certain policies and feels slighted by the apparent lack of service. The business may never know that the customer feels slighted.

- **The gap between members' expectations of service quality and actual performance.** The problems that exist if this gap occurs are quite obvious. If you do not know what your members expect of you and you give them something completely different, or even slightly different, you can be sure they will not be satisfied. You must do everything possible to learn what your members expect of you and then deliver it to their satisfaction.

- **The gap between marketing promises and actual delivery.** Many times a club promises to deliver a certain level of service quality and is unable to meet that promise. Making the promise has raised the level of expectation of the member (see the preceding bullet), and then not delivering on it has created an unhappy member. The simplest way to close this gap is to underpromise and overdeliver.

Closing these gaps is critical to your success in satisfying and retaining members. An important point to remember is that the member's perception of the situation is more important than your own until you can agree on a course of action together. Following are 10 questions you can ask to help you close these gaps and prevent them from occurring in the first place:

1. Have you asked your members what they need, want, and expect from you?

2. Is your club committed to providing superior service quality based on your member research?

3. Do you have a clear idea of how your members make purchase decisions?

4. Do you know what criteria your members use to define quality and to determine whether they are satisfied?

5. Have you overpromised on your service quality delivery capabilities?

6. Do your members perceive that you can meet their needs and expectations?

7. Do you understand your members' needs and expectations?

8. Do you have a performance measurement system in place to help identify member needs, wants, requirements, and expectations?

9. Do you have a recovery program in place to satisfy a dissatisfied member or to recapture a lost member?

10. Do your standards of service quality performance and customer satisfaction match your members' perceptual standards?

You can probably add several more questions to this list from your own experiences. These 10 will serve as an introductory guide for you as you attempt to close the service quality gaps that may exist and retain more of your members longer.

Inspecting What You Expect

You must set standards of performance, inform your staff and your members of those standards, and then measure your actual performance against those standards. When you set goals for your business based on your members' requirements and expectations, and then you publicly measure your performance toward those goals, you will have an excellent chance of improving both your service and level of member retention. The improvement comes from knowing where you are compared to where you want to be or should be and then taking the steps, based on the measurements, to improve your performance. Because your standards were developed in conjunction with customer perceptions, your meeting or exceeding those standards, as well as falling short, will give you a good indicator of how satisfied your customers will be and what you must do in the future.

Improved Performance Leads to Increased Profits

Although there is no guarantee that this will occur, it is a safe assumption that if you improve your service performance and delivery, you will probably benefit from increased profits. More people will want to buy from you, thereby increasing your volume contribution to profits. In other words, more people will want to join your club, buy from your pro shop, and refer others to you. Also, as your service performance improves and customer satisfaction levels increase, you can conceivably charge more money for your programs and services.

Learning How You Are Doing and Where to Go From Here

There are many very good reasons to measure your service quality performance and member satisfaction levels. This one may be the most important of all. Although you must find out what gaps exist and how to close them, and what your members need and expect and how they perceive the world, you need to know how you are doing right here, right now. Plus, you must be able to gather information on what you should be doing in the future. Member research will provide you with this information. Members will tell you if you are satisfying them now and what you must do to satisfy them in the future. They will also tell you whether you need to change your business strategy and/or business direction. Measuring members' perceptions of service quality and satisfaction levels is essential to your club's success.

Applying the Process of Continuous Improvement

No club can exist for long without continuously working to improve. If you do not try to continuously improve your service offerings, some other club will, and then your members will become their members. You must measure everything you do in order to improve. Ask your members as well as your employees how you can be better at what you do. Take their answers, suggestions, and recommendations and implement them within your club. Then ask again, and again, and again. Keep making those incremental improvements.

Remember that your goal is to establish long-term relationships with satisfied members. You do this by understanding and identifying their needs, meeting and exceeding their expectations, closing or removing any perceptual gaps that may exist between what you believe was delivered and what members believe was received, and trying to continuously improve your service quality efforts a little bit at a time.

The Benefits of Measuring Quality and Customer Satisfaction

The primary benefit of a measurement program is that it provides people with immediate, meaningful, and objective feedback. They can see how they are doing right now, compare it to some standard of excellence or performance, and decide what they must do to improve on that measurement. Have you ever asked yourself why basketball is so popular? It is because the player knows immediately if he or she succeeded. The player's performance is measured by whether the ball goes through the basket, and the player is motivated to try again. This motivation occurs regardless of whether the shot was successful.

Measurement provides people with a sense of accomplishment and a feeling of achievement. Measurements can also form the basis for a reward system that can only be successful if it is based on objective and quantifiable data. How will you know which employees or work teams to reward for improving quality and increasing customer satisfaction if you cannot, or do not, measure their performance?

These five items highlight the benefits of measuring customer satisfaction:

1. Measurement provides employees with a sense of achievement and accomplishment, which will then be translated into superior service to customers.

2. Measurement provides employees with a baseline standard of performance and a possible standard of excellence that they must try to achieve, which will lead to improved quality and increased customer satisfaction.

3. Measurement offers an employee immediate feedback, especially when the member is doing the measuring.

4. Measurement tells you what you must do to improve quality and customer satisfaction and how you must do it. This information can also come directly from the customer.

5. Measurement motivates employees to improve performance and achieve higher levels of productivity.

A Final Thought on Measuring Customer Satisfaction

Many club owners think that the improvements they make in customer service have to be small and incremental. They think that's the only way to increase customer satisfaction. However, I want to tell you from experience and common sense that if you have the chance to make a quantum leap in any performance area to increase customer satisfaction, do it. Don't ever get locked into the mind-set that you must do things a little bit at a time. If the situation presents itself for a major breakthrough in service performance related

> *Measurement provides people with a sense of accomplishment and a feeling of achievement.*

to customer/member satisfaction, go for it. Also, teach your employees, associates, and partners to go for it. When the big jump presents itself, jump!

There you have it. These are some of the most important reasons why you must measure quality and customer satisfaction. Now, I am going to discuss how to do it. The research techniques associated with measuring member satisfaction will be presented so that you do not have to be a statistician or an engineer to use them. In fact, I am neither, so I promise to present them in a manner everyone can understand.

Research Methods for Customer Satisfaction, Retention, and Loyalty

There are two types of data you can collect: primary and secondary. Both primary and secondary data collection techniques are valid as you try to measure your customers' satisfaction levels.

Secondary data is information you get from other sources not directly related to your club. Examples would be industry surveys on membership retention that are conducted by professional associations or trade groups. Another example of secondary data is when you apply experimental research findings to your club's operation. The advantages of secondary data are that it saves both money and time. The information is already available, and it is usually free, especially if you check your local library.

> **Member retention is the result of superior service performance and high levels of member satisfaction.**

The disadvantages are that the data may not directly fit your situation, the data may be obsolete by the time you use it, and the data may not be accurate enough for you to make informed decisions about your customer service and customer satisfaction work.

Primary data is information you collect yourself that is directly related to your measures of member satisfaction. Although primary data collection is much more accurate, because it relates specifically to the research you are conducting, it is also much more expensive. You collect primary data through a number of means, including but not limited to experiments, surveys, questionnaires, interviews, and opinion polls. You also use primary data to determine members' attitudes, opinions, preferences, behavior, and personalities. Plus, you (or one of your staff members) must invest a considerable amount of time into this effort.

You can use primary data collection to classify your current members into their demographic, psychographic, and sociographic categories. This classification helps you to more accurately determine the marketing and service approaches you want to take with these people. Furthermore, primary data will allow you to go even deeper and begin to service each member based on his or her individual preferences.

Qualitative Research

Qualitative research attempts to subjectively understand the experience of members when they join your club and participate in your programs. There are no hard measurements with qualitative research. You collect information on members' satisfaction levels through observation, interviews, focus groups, and personal experience, where you act as your own customer. (Have you ever called your own club to see how your employees respond?)

Even though you cannot quantify this type of information, you can gain tremendous insight into what your members think about your service, your programs, and your club. Usually, they will be more than happy to tell you their perceptions, thoughts, and feelings. You must then compile and collate this information so that you can use it to determine ways to improve your service and customer satisfaction ratings and increase retention.

Quantitative Research

Quantitative research is objective and measurable. You collect information according to some predetermined standard, such as a five- or seven-point scale, by using a questionnaire or survey. This survey can be written, asked face-to-face, or conducted over the telephone. When you have completed your research, you perform statistical analyses on the data to determine your customer satisfaction ratings.

Data Collection Techniques

You now have a basic background in research methods (for summary, see table 8.1). You are ready to develop your customer satisfaction research tools. I recommend you consider using one of these data collection techniques. If you look closely, they can all be considered subsets of a survey.

Questionnaires

Written surveys

Telephone surveys

Focus groups

Interviews (scheduled and personal)

Most customer satisfaction measurements are taken by surveys. These can be written or oral questionnaires, telephone or face-to-face interviews, and focus groups. The key is to get your members to respond and then for you to be able to use the data appropriately. Surveys usually consist of several questions and/or statements along with their associated responses that require people to answer according to some predefined scale. Some surveys allow people to answer in an open-ended manner, thereby describing their responses in greater detail. Both response methods are useful and provide excellent information about customer satisfaction levels.

TABLE 8.1 *Research Methods*

	Secondary Data	Primary Data	Qualitative Research	Quantitative Research
Definition	Information you get from sources not directly related to your club	Information you collect that is directly related to your measures of member satisfaction	Attempts to subjectively understand the experience of members joining club and participating in programs	Information collected according to a predetermined standard
Examples	Industry surveys or membership retention Experimenal research findings	Experiments Surveys Questionnaires Interviews Opinion polls	Observation Interviews Focus groups Personal experience	Written or telephone surveys Face-to-face interviews
Advantages	Save time and money Information readily available Free	Data can be used to classify members in demographic, psychographic, and sociographic categories Accurate	Gain tremendous insight	Objective and measurable
Disadvantages	Data may not directly fit situation Data may be obsolete by the time of use Data may not be accurate enough to make informed decisions	More expensive Requires considerable effort	No hard measurements Information must be compiled and collated to gain usable data	Statistical analyses require some effort

From these techniques, you can analyze the data to determine the following measurement and customer satisfaction reporting systems:

Service quality measurement system

Customer satisfaction index or rating

Customer report card

Service standards of performance

Customer satisfaction benchmarking

Attribute ratings and perceptual maps

The following sections provide a more detailed description of these reporting mechanisms.

Service Quality Measurement System (SQMS)

Your SQMS is the entire collection of tools and techniques you use to gather data and information about how well you are satisfying your customers. These tools can be any or all of the ones mentioned previously plus mystery shoppers or simple comment cards (which are actually mini-surveys). The system should be designed to alert you to areas the members think are important so that you can develop and implement programs to improve your services in those areas. Remember that you must ask the members again about your improvements to determine whether they are satisfied after you have made changes.

A problem with an SQMS is that it sometimes does not measure the types of service the member expects in order to be satisfied. It measures what the club thinks should be measured. This gap occurs when a club creates the entire system without asking and listening to the member. Before you prepare your satisfaction measurement tools and techniques, speak with your members and find out how they define quality, customer service, customer satisfaction, and anything else they can evaluate you on. Then, devise the SQMS to measure these things.

Customer/Member Satisfaction Index (CSI)

It can become very difficult for you to keep track of all the customer service, performance, and satisfaction data you collect. Therefore, you probably will find it easier to develop a customer satisfaction index or rating. This index is usually a compilation of your scores into one number or percentage. For example, if you have members rate you on 50 items or factors related to their satisfaction, you can take an average of all those scores and call it your index. Or you can weight the responses according to importance and then create an index from the weighted scores. However you do it, remember that the CSI is not an individual rating but an average or compilation of many ratings.

Customer/Member Report Card

This simple approach quickly determines how customers feel about certain attributes related to the service you are providing. Many companies use a comment card to serve as a report card. Your club can do the same thing; it is quick and easy.

You develop the customer report card by first asking members what attributes of your service they consider when they are determining their satisfaction levels. You then place these attributes on a comment card and ask the members to rate them according to some scale. You analyze the scores and data from these brief surveys the same way you would from more extensive surveys. An advantage of a customer report card is that it is short, easy to fill out, and easy to score. Your report card rating can be a numerical total of all the ratings made by the customers or a letter grade, much like your child's report card in school. Figure 8.1 shows an example.

XYZ HEALTH AND FITNESS CLUB APPRECIATES YOUR COMMENTS

Cleanliness	Excellent	Good	Fair	Poor	Very bad
Locker rooms	Excellent	Good	Fair	Poor	Very bad
Instructors	Excellent	Good	Fair	Poor	Very bad
Courtesy of staff	Excellent	Good	Fair	Poor	Very bad
Prices	Excellent	Good	Fair	Poor	Very bad
Professionalism of staff	Excellent	Good	Fair	Poor	Very bad
Personal trainers	Excellent	Good	Fair	Poor	Very bad

FIGURE 8.1 *A sample customer report card*

You can see from figure 8.1 that a club can quickly get a picture of how well it is servicing its members. To analyze the ratings, you can assign numbers to each verbal descriptor; for example, Excellent could be a 5 and Very bad could be a 1. Then you just have to add up the scores to get an overall rating for the club. You can also average the scores within specific rating categories to determine which areas need the most attention.

Service Standards of Performance (SOPs)

Service standards of performance have more to do with your employees than with your customers, yet service SOPs are vitally important to your success in improving service and customer satisfaction. Although service is an intangible, and quite often a customer's level of satisfaction is highly subjective, some employee behaviors are measurable. It is these behaviors that you quantify as the service standards of performance.

Examples of SOPs include answering the telephone before the fourth ring, saying the member's name at least once if you know it, always saying thank you to a member, resolving complaints in a timely fashion and to the member's satisfaction, responding to members within 30 seconds after they enter your facility, returning all telephone calls within 24 hours, responding to all correspondence within 24 hours, keeping a member's waiting time under 5 minutes, and completing a purchase or exchange transaction within a certain period of time. These are all possible objective standards of performance you can use.

One thing you must remember about service SOPs. You are rating your employees on their abilities to service and satisfy your customers. When the employees receive high ratings from you or your customers, the employees should be rewarded so these behaviors are reinforced. Service SOPs without an employee reward and recognition program will not help you improve your service quality and levels of customer satisfaction because employees will not feel that their efforts are appreciated.

Customer Satisfaction Benchmarking

Traditional benchmarking is a method to measure how well you are doing compared to other clubs and other businesses outside the fitness industry. Benchmarking is simply finding a company that is the best at something and comparing your efforts in the same area. You then adapt and modify that company's work or approach to fit your situation and improve your service, job performance, and programs. The goal is to increase your member satisfaction and retention as a result of these improvement efforts.

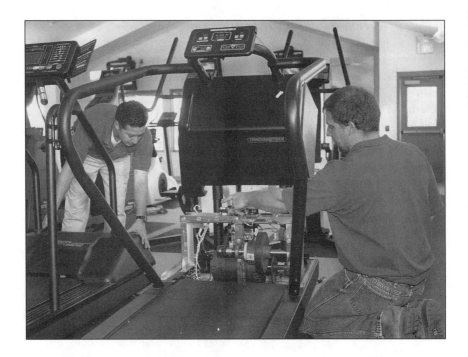

Customer satisfaction benchmarking works the same way. Find a company, either in or out of your industry, that consistently receives high satisfaction ratings. Find out what it does in each area and how it does it and how it measures customer satisfaction, and then adapt its techniques to your club. Constant comparisons with the "best in class" will force you to improve your service and job performance, which results in an increase in levels of customer satisfaction.

Also, never forget about internal benchmarking. You should consistently measure the satisfaction levels of your customers and use each subsequent measurement as the benchmark for future measurements. This way, you have a basis for ongoing comparison within your own company.

Attribute Ratings and Perceptual Maps

Many times, members unknowingly compare one service attribute of your club with another, or they compare it with the same attribute from a competitor's business. Suppose you provide in-home personal training for your members, and you pride yourself on having a trainer at a member's home within 10 minutes of the appointed time. This timeliness is one of your service attributes. Now, members can compare this attribute with the quality of the workout your trainer provides or with the speed/availability of a competitor's trainer. Or they can trade off the quality of the workout with the friendliness of the trainer. As another outside example, in a restaurant, customers may compare how food looks (the presentation attribute) with how it tastes.

You find out what attributes your members are using to evaluate your service performance by asking them or reviewing your written and personal surveys to determine which key service areas keep coming up. Then, you can focus on those key areas so that when you measure the service attributes, you are doing well in the members' minds.

There are many ways to measure satisfaction based on service attributes. You can ask customers to rank several key attributes in order of importance to them. You can ask them what they like best about what you do and then how important that attribute is to them. You can ask them to compare your performance on certain service attributes with the performance of other clubs. Or if these attributes are similar to businesses in other industries, you can have the members compare you to their other service experiences.

You now have several ways to measure your service performance and customer satisfaction. The key is to develop these procedures and use them on a regular basis. Member retention is the result of superior service performance and high levels of member satisfaction. Member loyalty comes from your long-term members who totally believe in what you are doing for them. It's a very simple chain that links service with satisfaction, retention, and then loyalty. You must follow the path in this order so that you keep the links strong. Remember that improvements in service performance will lead to increases in customer satisfaction, which will result in greater retention of members and an increase in their loyalty to your club.

CHAPTER 9

Customer Service as a Powerful Marketing and Retention Tool

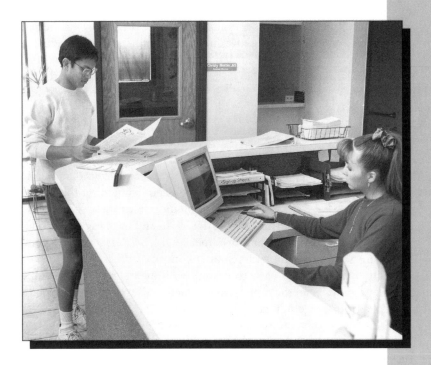

You're probably already implementing a number of excellent marketing tactics to improve your member retention, and you may not even know it. For example, if you send out a club newsletter, that's a marketing approach that can lead to increased member retention. If you have special programs just for members, that will lead to increased retention. If you send out birthday cards or congratulations notices for job promotions, that's relationship and retention marketing at its finest. If you call up a member who has not been in for a while, or go see a sick member at home or in the hospital, you are promoting member retention. In fact, anything you do to consistently communicate with members and show them you care helps to build member retention.

Remember that member retention is not primarily about programming. It's about getting into the hearts and minds of your members. It's about becoming a part of their lifestyles and their lives. Retention has to do with how well your employees treat the members as people more than how many programs you run each month.

If a member leaves your club, do you call up to try to save the membership by offering special incentives or discounts, or are you more interested in the member's personal reasons for leaving? Although saving the membership is important, I believe it's more important to treat the former member as a person. When you show you care about the member as an individual, and are truly interested in why he or she left instead of trying to win the member back, you may be surprised with the results of your efforts. Former members may come back on their own, and their commitment to you will be stronger than ever.

> **People want to belong to a club that delivers on its promises and honors its guarantees.**

Only in the past several years have club owners realized that member service is not something that is done to a member, but rather something that is done for a member. During most of the 1980s and the early part of the 1990s, owners perceived member and customer service more as a reactive, complaint-handling activity to deal with member concerns and problems rather than a proactive, positive approach to dealing with members. Finally, club owners began to understand the importance of member service in the marketing mix and the significance of relationship and retention marketing.

Clubs across the country have learned that when they are proactive with their member service efforts, they will acquire and keep customers more easily and for longer periods of time. Members are now drawn to clubs that clearly communicate their service message. What separates one club from another is very often the level of customer service provided to its members. After all, equipment is equipment and furniture/fixtures are furniture/fixtures. So the difference between clubs that easily acquire and keep their members and clubs that don't must be in the actual and perceived level of customer service.

Here's another example of how to use member service and guarantees as a marketing tool to get and keep members for life. Several years ago, I was asked to work with a club that was spending a great deal of money to advertise for memberships. The reason was that their attrition rate was over 60 percent.

When you combine high member acquisition costs with high attrition rates, you will never have a profitable club. You can be sure that this club wasn't profitable; several problems had to be corrected.

I began by interviewing the current members, then by calling the lapsed members and asking them what was good, bad, or indifferent about the club. When I talked with former members, certain major problems kept coming up. "No one on the staff cared about the members as people." "The club just seemed to want to sell memberships without doing anything for the members, and they took my money and never delivered anything they promised." Does this sound familiar? When I had these answers, I began working on the club's marketing approach.

Here are just a few of the things the club management and I did. First, we contacted all the lapsed members and offered them a free three-month membership to try out the "new" club. We made specific service promises to them and then guaranteed we would deliver on them. We also extended the three-day "cooling-off" period to 30 days for new members. These guarantees showed them that we believed in the club and what we could provide.

We also changed the advertising to reflect these newly developed service promises and promoted the extended guarantee. We decided to spend less on the advertising and more on internal promotions to generate member referrals. Then, we repeatedly surveyed the members to find out what they needed, wanted, and expected, and then we delivered. In one year, attrition rates dropped to 25 percent, new member acquisition costs decreased by 30 percent, and the advertising costs decreased by 50 percent. More new members came into the club than ever before, lapsed members tried the three-month free trial and then signed up again, and the majority of these people stayed on for an additional year (or more).

The purpose of this story is to show you how member service can be used as a powerful marketing tool, when it is properly promoted. Think of a way you can apply some of these ideas to your club. Plus, think of things from the perspective of your members. What type of club do they want to belong to? They want to belong to a club that delivers on its promises and honors its guarantees.

In the rest of this chapter, I'm going to describe for you what I consider to be some of the best member service and retention marketing techniques you can use to build your club. Now, if you're wondering what member service has to do with marketing, just ask yourself how members decide what makes you different from your competitors and why they should buy from you. Their decisions are based on the information they receive from your marketing communications. My files are full of case studies that support the use of any or all of these techniques for building a club or a business in any other industry.

Putting Ideas to Use

The following sections explain how to use these member service and retention marketing techniques to build your club. When you hit on the right combination of these techniques for your specific club, you can double your club revenues in 12 months or less without any other marketing efforts.

Frequent Buyer Programs

Frequent buyer programs are similar to the frequent flier programs promoted by the airlines. When you fly often enough and far enough with any given airline, you receive mileage credits that can be turned in for free tickets, ticket upgrades, or even free vacations. The more you fly, the more credits you receive.

You set up the same type of program in your club for your members. The purpose of the frequent buyer program is to show your members how much you appreciate their business. The more they buy from you, either in the form of number of memberships or purchases in your pro shop, the more you give back to them. You reward your best members for continuing to buy from you on a regular basis.

Make sure it's easy for all your members to be part of this program. Keep track of their purchases in your database program so you can identify who gets what type of reward. Then, give them something that keeps them coming back for more. How you reward them is not as important as the fact that you do reward them. (As you'll see in the next section on frequent referral programs, your rewards don't have to be expensive. They just have to have a high perceived value in the member's mind.)

Frequent Referral Programs

The club industry thrives on referrals, as does any other business. Clubs have special promotions (member-get-a-member programs and so on), special days, free guest passes, and a whole host of other things they do to generate member referrals. Probably the most effective tool is to create a frequent referral program. This program rewards members who refer new members to the club. The rewards can be T-shirts, caps, free personal training, court time, extensions on memberships, and anything else you can think of. The important thing is to recognize the member's efforts and to reward them accordingly.

You can create what I call a tiered reward program, where the gifts or incentives you provide increase in value as the number of member referrals increases. First, use your membership database to track the number of referrals provided by each member. When the member reaches a certain level, give the member an appropriate reward. Some examples include a T-shirt for one referral in a given month, a workout bag for three referrals, and free personal training for five referrals. Then, you can start the process all over again. Or you can extend their membership for free for every new member they refer or bring through your door. I even suggest that when someone refers 10 new members to your club, you should send that person on a cruise. Just remember to recognize those members that refer new members to you. This recognition motivates them to continue to market on your behalf, and there is no up-front cost to you. You now have the most motivated unpaid sales force in the world.

Thank-You Cards

"Thank-you" are two of the most cherished, powerful words in any language, yet they are never used enough. Here's your opportunity to turn two simple words into a powerful marketing tool. Just remember to say "thank-you" to members for every purchase they make, every referral they provide, and anything else they do that involves your club or staff. Also, send handwritten thank-you cards to members after they join, to prospects who come in and take a tour, and to vendors you use.

The few extra minutes you spend writing the thank-you cards will more than pay for themselves in future business. Although writing and sending thank-you cards seems so simple, people really appreciate them because so few people take the time to send them. Sending a handwritten thank-you note elevates your status in the recipient's mind. I've received training contracts from clients because I took the time to send them a thank-you note when other people couldn't be bothered.

Cards show you care.

Here's a twist on the typical thank-you card. I've used it very successfully, and it makes my company stand out in the minds of the many clients I have. It will make your club stand out also if you use this approach or a variation of it. I've created a thank-you card on a plastic credit card that says "Thank-you for . . ." The sentence ends with either meeting with me; your business; or your referral. These three messages get my thank-you across to the prospect or client.

What makes these cards even more memorable is that they are prepaid, discounted phone cards that offer the recipient five minutes of free long-distance phone time. Imagine the position that you'll hold in your members' minds if you give them free long-distance calling whenever you say thank-you. (The cost to purchase the phone time and the card is very inexpensive.) Plus, because the cards are plastic, the recipients keep them in their wallets. So every time the recipients use a card to make a call, your club's name is right there in front of them.

Holiday and Birthday Cards

If you think I'm card-crazy, you're right. People love to receive cards in the mail. It gives them such a positive feeling to know someone is thinking of them at a special time. It's even more uplifting and surprising if those cards come from a club associate, from whom it's unexpected, rather than a family member or friend. Cards show you care.

I strongly recommend you send holiday cards to all your members. These can be Thanksgiving, Hanukkah, Christmas, New Year's, or whenever cards. If you're worried about your cards getting lost in the holiday mail, send them out early, like around the 4th of July or Halloween. Sure, it's way before your members might expect it, but that's the point. It's so unexpected that they'll remember you for it.

The same is true for birthday cards. If you can get the birth dates of your members (and you should have them in your database from their initial application), they'll be pleasantly surprised to receive a birthday card from you. It's a simple and inexpensive gesture on your part, and it takes little of your time. Yet the payoff in additional purchases and referrals that you'll receive from this action is tremendous.

One word of caution: Never, ever send anniversary cards to someone. You never know if that person has gotten separated or divorced since the last time you had contact with them. Although this may seem like a minor point, I strongly suggest you stay away from anniversary cards. You can do what you want. It's your club. I'm just telling you that you shouldn't take this type of chance.

I don't want to end this section on a gloomy note, so here's a way to extend the holiday card idea. Give holiday gifts to your members. Again, these gifts don't have to be expensive. They just should have a perceived value in the minds of the members. Now, you may be saying that you have hundreds or thousands (or will one day have) of members, and this idea can get expensive. You're right; it can become expensive. But how much is that member worth to you? How much revenue does that member bring to you each year? Isn't he or she worth a $5, $10, or $25 gift to show you appreciate his or her business? What other club do you know of that offers its members holiday gifts? If you're the first and only, you'll stand out as the place to join to get in shape.

Reward and Recognition Programs

You must do everything possible to recognize and reward your members and employees. Sending them cards shows them you care and that you recognize their contributions to your business, but you still must do something else. Make a big deal out of how you recognize someone. People love to be made to feel important, so do what you can to elevate their self-esteem. Build them up verbally and in writing. Then when you create your reward programs, make sure the rewards are psychologically satisfying to the recipients.

Many clubs I've dealt with, and companies in other industries, think that money is always the answer as a reward. It's not. Sometimes, T-shirts, gift certificates, membership extensions, time off for employees, trips, and so on are more valuable to a person than money. You may be surprised to learn that some of your members can't accept money for anything because of regulations or laws. The best way to identify the most effective rewards is to ask the people who one day will be receiving them. Find out what they like and then give it to them.

Another thing that all club employees must do is learn the names of all the members and use those names properly and often. A person's name correctly coming off someone else's lips is the sweetest sound in the world to that person. Train your staff to learn and memorize members' names, and the members will love you for it. Plus, remembering a member's name

> *Recognize members' efforts and reward them accordingly.*

makes that person feel important. The more important your members feel, the more likely they are to stay with you for the long term. This action alone may be enough of a reward for some of your members. Especially if people constantly misspell or mispronounce their name and your staff says it correctly all the time.

When you recognize and reward your members and employees, you create a psychological allegiance that makes it difficult for them to switch to another club. Many times, it is the perceived psychological switching costs, rather than prices or program fees, that keeps a member with one club. Use your recognition and reward programs to increase the perceived value of a person's membership. The result will be more members staying with you longer.

Recall and Reactivation Programs

Of all the great ways to use member service as a powerful marketing tool, this technique can generate more revenue for your club than several of the other techniques combined. Reactivating your old members can create new revenue streams you never thought possible. From a pure marketing perspective, this technique is one way to deploy hidden assets. I call them hidden because most club owners stop paying attention to them and forget they exist. If you need any motivation to implement this type of program, just remember that it costs five to six times more to get a new member than it does to get an old member to rejoin.

One club owner I worked with kept careful records of all the club's members. The club had a membership base of about 1,500 and was losing 75 members a month. I suggested that the club try a reactivation program based on its database. I had the computer flag members whose membership had lapsed 90 days ago. The club sent them a letter inviting them to come back to the club. Attached to the letter was a coupon for a free personal training session.

This approach reactivated 45 percent of the 225 members it was sent to within 30 days. If the average annual membership fee is $400, then this club brought in an additional $40,000 or so just by reactivating old members. Plus, the club owner began to survey these returning members to find out why they left in the first place. The feedback was then used to make improvements in the operation of the club and the member service.

As a speaker, trainer, and consultant, I call up former clients (one year old) to see how they are doing and to ask if there is anything I can help them with. I call this my "Hello, how are you?" call because it is not a direct sales call. It's just a friendly reminder that I'm still around and interested in helping them achieve their goals. Although not everyone responds immediately, I do get several calls for additional work. Sometimes these calls come in a few weeks, other times they come a few months later. One campaign alone generated over $20,000 in revenue in two months from former clients.

This "Hello, how are you?" call to former members is wonderful for re-establishing the rapport and trust that you once had and for motivating them to do business with you again. This approach becomes even more powerful if you don't sound as though you're asking for their business while you're on the phone. Remember that they don't care how much you know until they know how much you care. Show them you care by talking about them and their needs, wants, and problems instead of trying to get them to rejoin.

Think of the sheer magnitude and potential of this concept. There are no acquisition costs; no time is required to build trust and rapport; no energy investment is necessary to prove yourself; and there's no interference from competitors. Just a simple phone call or letter asking your former members how they are, what's doing in their personal and professional lives, and possibly offering them something for free just to come in to see you, sending them a small gift to show your appreciation for their past business, or just doing something for them that they didn't expect of you. All these actions on your part show former members that you still care about them, that they are still important to you, and that you appreciate them as people and members.

Another twist on the recall concept is confirmation calls. Whenever a member has an appointment in your club, with a personal trainer for example, you call that member 24 hours in advance to remind him or her of the appointment. It took a while for some professionals to accept this type of retention marketing approach, but I'll bet you that your doctor's office or dentist's office calls you to remind you of your appointments. That member will appreciate your thoughtfulness and the effort you are making on their behalf.

Many businesses send a preprinted thank-you note (very impersonal) or make an obligatory phone call (you can hear the obligation in the caller's voice) after a member makes a purchase. Unfortunately, these efforts are superficial at best. You can stand out from the crowd by calling everyone who buys from you, sincerely thanking them for their purchase, and promising to help them achieve their fitness goals in every way possible.

Members often experience dissonance or feelings of uncertainty or uneasiness after a purchase, especially an expensive one. You know it as buyer's remorse. It's when you, and they, start to question themselves: Did I make the right choice? Did I really need to spend all that money? Should I have visited other clubs? Will this club deliver on its promises?

You know exactly what I'm talking about because you and I have also gone through it. Do you think an obligatory card or call will resolve the dissonance issue? No way. You need to make a post-purchase reassurance phone call and sincerely tell members that they made the right choice in purchasing the membership from you. Reassure them that you'll always be available to provide them with the service you've promised and that they've come to expect from you. Then follow up this call with a letter saying the same thing. Doing this will separate you from the competition and will create loyal members who will stay with you and refer others to you. Doing this may also prevent you from having to develop a recall and reactivation program because your members are staying with you instead of leaving you.

Satisfaction Guaranteed (Risk Reversal)

Everyone in business today is offering some sort of guarantee. If they are not, they should be. A satisfaction guarantee has become the standard for getting people to buy from you. You see or hear of these guarantees all the time:

"Satisfaction guaranteed or your money back."

"Full refund in 30 days with your receipt. Otherwise, a credit for a future purchase or an exchange will be issued."

"90-day, money-back guarantee."

"Try the first issue free. If you don't like the magazine, write cancel on the invoice and send it back. The first issue is yours to keep."

These are just some of the ways companies offer guarantees to satisfy customers. Guarantees are based on the psychological concept of risk reversal. Risk reversal means doing whatever it takes to remove as much of the psychological and financial burden of purchasing from the member.

Guarantees are great, and you should offer them. People want extra value for every dollar they spend. They want to be assured that they are getting exactly what they're paying for and more. The 72-hour cooling-off period after purchasing a membership is like a guarantee. Can you extend this period to set your club apart from the others? Check out your competition to see whether they're offering any guarantees on memberships. If they are, figure out how you can go them one better. If they're not offering any type of guarantee, you've got a great opportunity.

You can also provide a better-than-risk-free guarantee. Let people know that when they purchase a membership from you, they get what they buy plus a small gift from you. If they decide they're not happy with the membership and they cancel it, they still get to keep the gift. The gift can be an engraved coffee mug with the club's logo and name on it, a club workout towel, or a coupon for three free personal training sessions. What you give is not as important as the perception it activates in the member's mind.

What you've done here is totally reverse the risk of purchasing. You've taken the burden of the decision off the shoulders of the buyer and placed it squarely on your own shoulders. Plus, you've placed a thought in the buyer's mind about how confident you are in your club's capability to deliver on the promises made during the sale of the membership. After all, would anyone other than a highly confident provider offer a gift with the membership purchase, knowing that the member can cancel and still keep the gift?

Think of situations where you bought something from a catalog company or in a department store, especially around the holiday time. You always get a gift with the purchase that you can keep, even if you return the purchase. The same is true with many magazines. Although this type of guarantee should make you feel very comfortable buying from these companies, you're probably wondering how you can apply this to your club. Plus, you may be concerned about people who will take advantage of your guarantee. Let me put your fears aside.

First, applying the risk reversal concept to your club is easy. Just offer a standard guarantee that's better than your competitors and then give members a small gift in addition to the purchase. Let the members know they can cancel their membership at any time if they're not satisfied, and you'll refund their money. You can set standards for the cancellation and make sure members adhere to those standards, if you want to. But this does detract from your guarantee, and members can still keep the gift they received when they joined.

To really put some power into a guarantee related to the cooling-off period, extend the cooling-off period from the typical three days after purchasing a membership to 30, 60, or 90 days or even a full year. If the members are ever dissatisfied, you'll take care of them. You'll give them their money back, you'll extend their membership, or you'll do whatever it takes to satisfy them. Although this may sound like a big risk on your part, realize that only 2 to 5 percent of your members will take advantage of your guarantee. The rest will be happy with your service and stay with you. Run the club for the 95 to 98 percent of the satisfied members. Besides, if a member is truly dissatisfied with your club, would you really want that person running around your club complaining to other members about their perception of your service?

To me, the answer is a no-brainer. Do whatever it takes, within reason, to guarantee the purchase and satisfaction of your members. In my business, people who purchase my books and tapes directly from me have a lifetime guarantee. If, for any reason, they are ever dissatisfied with their purchase, they can return it to me for a full refund or credit. The only stipulation is that the products are in resalable condition, which means I have to be able to repackage them and sell them to another customer. If the products don't meet the resalable condition criteria, then the customers can't return the items. Also, if someone buys products from me and then returns them, and does this three different times, that person is put on a "do not ship" list because I know he or she is just copying my products and then returning them for a refund.

Offer a satisfaction guarantee to your members, and then go beyond that by reversing the risk of purchasing as much as possible. Your ultimate risk reversal is in adapting some of the previous methods of offering the better-than-risk-free guarantee. When you communicate this policy to members and prospects, people will flock to join your club.

Guarantees (and warranties) are more often associated with manufactured products, but the club owner who develops an ironclad membership or service guarantee and promotes it will stand out from the competition. Therein lies one of the keys to success when using service guarantees as a marketing tool. If you have one, but no one knows about it (that is, you haven't communicated it through your marketing efforts), it will not help you attract members. You must market and promote your program, service, and member guarantees. Those clubs that do so will acquire members more easily and at a lower cost.

For example, if your club is promoting a weight-loss program, and you have several members join for a charge over and above their membership fees, you could entice more people to join by guaranteeing your results. Just require the participants to keep an accurate log of their workouts and food consumption, and then if for some reason they don't lose the desired weight, give them their money back for the program. You will rarely have to refund money. But in the few instances that you do, the fact that you live up to your guarantee will become a powerful marketing message to your current and future members.

The guarantee works as a retention marketing tool because the risk of the purchase is transferred from the member to the club. When potential members have little or no risk associated with joining your club or purchasing add-on programs, then they are more likely to sign up and participate regularly. It's only after they feel comfortable and are seeing their desired results that their perceived risk decreases. So if you take the initial risk off their shoulders by offering an extended satisfaction guarantee, more people will join. Plus, when you deliver the level of service you promise, more people will stay with your club longer. What if you extended the typical 72-hour cooling-off period after a member joins to a week, a month, or even a whole year? What would that say about your confidence in your level of service?

Treating Employees as Customers

It is extremely important to recognize and reward your employees for out-standing service performances. If you've already established service standards of performance (and you should have), and your employees meet or exceed those standards, then you must reward them as you would your members for positive behaviors (such as referrals). This reward will motivate them to continue these positive behaviors.

Just as important is the fact that you must realize your employees are customers, too. They are your internal customers, and they must be treated with the courtesy and respect you provide to your buying members. Too often, I've worked with clubs that had customer service problems because management or the owners told the employees to provide great service to the members, yet the employees were treated like second-class citizens. Aside from the fact that little or no customer service training was provided, the employees were treated exactly the opposite of the way they were supposed to treat the members.

Do you remember the poem about children learning what they live and living what they learn? Adults are the same as children. You can't expect staff people to provide great service if you don't treat them with the same respect, courtesy, and professionalism you expect them to provide to members. How can any club owner expect employees to provide great member service if they are treated poorly? People are people, and they must be treated accordingly. Remember that your staff will treat members the way you treat your staff.

If you put your customers up on pedestals, put your employees up on pedestals too. If you'd never yell at a customer in public, or berate a member in public, don't do that to an employee either. If you'd never belittle a member's self-esteem, don't put down your employees either.

There's another philosophy related to treating employees as customers that states "The member comes second." This philosophy is in stark contrast to what many authors, consultants, and customer service experts would have us believe. We've always been told that the customer comes first. The customer is king (or queen). The customer is always right. However, the concept of the member coming second has merit for every club. The premise is that the employees come first in your, and any, company. When the employees are treated well, then they will treat the members well. Take care of your employees, and they will take care of your members and your club.

It's the same philosophy I recommend to everyone for their own personal development. Before you can take care of anyone else or help anyone else accomplish anything, you must first take care of yourself and help yourself. You can't be any good to anyone else if you're not good to yourself first. The bottom line is that you must provide great service to your employees. They, in turn, will provide great service to your members. Then, the bottom line will become bigger.

Member Special Events

Every club, at one time or another, holds member functions. Special workout contests, socials, picnics, and so on are standard fare. You have to determine how your special events will be different. I don't mean more lavish or expensive. Just different enough so that the members perceive that you really went out of your way for them and they will remember what you did.

You can develop VIP programs, private parties for your best referral sources, day trips for your longest term members, and any number of other ideas you can come up with. Check out businesses in other industries and see what they are doing. Investigate your competition and see what they're doing. Find out how their members respond to their special events. Then, go them one better.

Do it bigger, louder, flashier, smaller, quieter, or funnier. Just do it and do it differently and better. The result will be members who will feel more special in your club than anywhere else. When you make members feel special and important, they will stay with you because you're reinforcing their positive self-image and self-esteem. (Never underestimate your role or power of influence in the situation of their psychological health and well-being.) You can also poll your members to determine what types of special events they like and are interested in participating in. When you give them what they want, they appreciate your consideration. Out of loyalty, they will stay with you longer.

There is one other benefit to these member special events. As your members network during these events, they will establish new business relationships that will help them be more successful on the job. They will be appreciative of your efforts on their behalf, and this appreciation will enhance their psychological loyalty to you. They will also reward you with more referrals.

Strategic Member Alliances

Do your best to form strong alliances with your members. Get them involved in member advisory councils and inspection programs where they inspect your club and tell you exactly what you need to do to improve and offer them commissions on referral sales (reward and recognition programs). Get with your longest term members and find out if they'll become club advocates. See whether they want to be ombudsmen for other members. Ask them if they want to form their own service council. The idea is to make members feel like partners in your club. Partners (not financial) perceive an obligation to do what's best for their business, and your member/partners will go out of their way to treat your club right.

An added benefit of involving your members in the operation of your club is that they will want to reciprocate your kindness. They'll do this by staying with you longer and referring more and more people to become members. Plus, they'll be saying positive things about you and your club to everyone they meet. You may even want to give your members business cards that say member representative on them. Just like your salespeople have cards with passes on the back, your members could have similar cards. They can pick and choose who they give these business cards to, but you can be sure when they do give one out, that the person is a highly qualified prospect for becoming a member.

Use these powerful customer service techniques as member retention marketing tools. You have all the information you need to make these techniques work right at your fingertips. Check your database. Shake hands with your members. Pat your staff members on the back. Every one of these fingertip activities will position you deeper in your members' minds. Their perceptions of you will continue to be positive. The psychological bond that

MEMBER RETENTION TECHNIQUES

- Frequent buyer programs
- Frequent referral programs
- Thank-you cards
- Holiday and birthday cards
- Reward and recognition programs
- Recall and reactivation programs
- Satisfaction guaranteed (risk reversal)
- Treating employees as customers
- Member special events
- Strategic member alliances

you create will become stronger. The results will be consistent growth in your club. Your bottom line will increase as your customer acquisition costs decrease and more members stay with you longer. The lifetime value of each member will increase and their profit contribution will increase. Who knows, you may even have to create a waiting list for memberships. Now, wouldn't that be a nice problem to have?

part three

Member Relationship Management (Keeping Members for Life)

CHAPTER 10

The Member Relationship Management Process

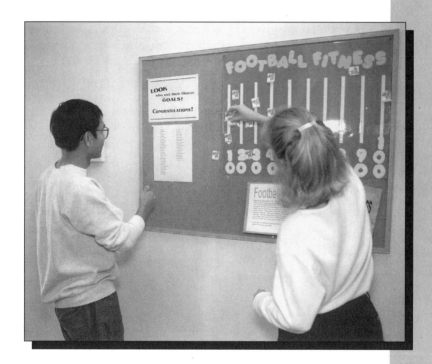

You and I both know that the old public image and impression of the health club industry is not true anymore. You remember that image: People believed that clubs only wanted their money, and once they got it, they wouldn't do anything to serve them as members. Clubs relied on *churn* to keep their money flowing without overloading the club. You also should remember the old statistic that said most of your members would stop using the club within 90 days, but they would keep paying. That's how the churn worked. You kept selling memberships regardless of the club's capacity because utilization would drop off and find its own level in your club.

But we both know that this is not the way it works anymore, is it? Maybe we're kidding ourselves. I have interviewed hundreds of club members from what I call the casual user category. These people use a club once a week or less. Over 75 percent of these people still believe the club is only interested in getting their money and is hoping they don't show up to use the facility. This way, the club can keep selling more memberships.

I recently spoke with the general manager of a club who told me he was having a difficult time meeting his sales goals. He needed to sell 110 memberships a month just to stay even because his attrition rate was 50 percent. You already know from previous chapters that you have to focus on retention more than new sales. It's a business concept. But this manager was so focused on new sales, he neglected his current membership base. Now, 55 members a month were leaving by either not renewing or by finding ways to get out of their contracts. He was at a loss for what to do.

I suggested we look at the entire membership experience in his club. I call it the member relationship process. I explained to him that every member has a finite life cycle with a club and that you must engage in certain activities during each phase of that cycle. When you complete the proper activities during the appropriate phase of the member's life cycle, you are going a long way to ensuring that the member becomes and stays loyal. When he relayed this information to his owner, he was told to forget about this retention philosophy and focus on selling more new memberships. Maybe the club image perceived by the casual member is really not so far off.

Everyone likes to be recognized for their achievements.

Anyway, let me introduce you to the member relationship management (MRM) process and a member's life cycle with your club. There are four phases to the process, and each phase has activities within. The phases are called CARE to make them easy to remember. The C is for contact, which involves all the ways you would contact a member or potential member. The A is for acquisition, and it covers the activities involved in making the sale and moving the member forward through the model. The R is for retention, which is what you must do to keep the member. Finally, the E is for extension, and it covers the areas related to loyalty, defection, and increased referrals.

There are also costs associated with each phase. During the Contact phase, you must consider all your marketing and advertising costs and the cost of sales. During the Acquisition phase, you must know your acquisition costs, your lost opportunity costs, and your costs related to poor service (these have been

FOUR PHASES OF THE MEMBER RELATIONSHIP MANAGEMENT (MRM) PROCESS

The phases are called CARE to make them easy to remember.

C is for contact, which involves all the ways you would contact a member or potential member.

A is for acquisition, and it covers the activities involved in making the sale and moving the member forward through the model.

R is for retention, which is what you must do to keep the member.

E is for extension, and it covers the areas related to loyalty, defection, and increased referrals.

described previously in this book). During the Retention phase, you must calculate your complaint costs, your service problem costs, and any incentive program costs. Finally, in the Extension phase, you must know your defection costs, your customer save costs (what it costs you to stop a customer from defecting), and your relationship costs (what you spend to maintain the relationship).

Throughout the rest of this chapter, I will describe the entire member relationship management process to you. I will cover each phase and its component activities, along with the related costs. I will also give you examples of how this process affects your club business, and why you must focus all of these activities on member retention.

The Contact Phase

The Contact phase is when you get in touch with your prospective member. It involves all your marketing, advertising, and sales activities, including direct mail, personal selling, telemarketing and telesales, e-mail, a web site, and any other methods you can think of to communicate with your target market.

The important point here is that you now make a distinction in your contact efforts. Traditionally, clubs advertised their programs and membership services in the most attractive manner possible. They were establishing customer expectations that many clubs could not, and did not meet. So when members joined, they were sorely disappointed that the club never lived up to its promises that it made in the advertising or marketing.

Take a long, hard look at your marketing and advertising. I urge you to consider revising your efforts to focus on the member and what you can do to keep that member over time. Let the member know that you're interested in him or her as a person, rather than a number or a "financier." When you do an ad in the newspaper, on radio, or on television, make it speak directly to your prospective member. Create the ad as if you were talking to them one on one. Appeal to their emotions and engage them as a whole person. Whatever promises you make in your advertising or marketing or during your sales presentation, make sure you can keep them during your service delivery.

Contact Costs

You must know your contact-related costs. These costs are more than your advertising or marketing budget. They're also more than what you spend to place the ads or send out the mail pieces. You must also include all your developmental costs, your production costs, and your sales costs. Plus, you should allocate some general and administrative expenses to your marketing efforts. This addition will give you a clearer picture of your contact costs, and it will also help you calculate your member acquisition costs, which is done in the next phase.

Many club owners that I've spoken with are unaware of the actual cost of acquiring a member. That's because they don't know what they spend to get a prospect in the door. You must be fully aware of all your prospecting, lead-generating, and marketing expenditures. That's the only way you'll be able to initially determine whether a member is financially profitable and worth keeping.

The Acquisition Phase

You must be aware of these seven areas during the Acquisition phase:

1. Your image and reputation
2. The first purchase conditions as perceived by the new member
3. The price/value perceptions of the member
4. The need state of the member
5. The foundation or basis for the relationship the member wishes to establish
6. Your post-purchase reassurance behaviors
7. Your guarantee or warranty

Let's look at each area individually, and then I'll discuss the costs associated with this stage.

Image/Reputation

I've already talked about the image and reputation that the club industry has in the minds of some consumers. Although those of us inside the industry know the steps we are taking to make this image more positive, outsiders (members) may be unaware of our efforts. That's why so many people still have a negative perception of the industry.

Ask yourself the following questions: What is your image to your current members? Is it positive? Are you friendly? Is your club clean? Is your club a leader in the field? What about your reputation? Do you do what you say you're going to do for members? Do you deliver on your promises? Do you do it on time? Do you solicit feedback from members to improve your club?

These questions are important to answer in order to make it easier to acquire new members. Your image is what you look, feel, smell, and taste like to the members. It's what they see and perceive with all their senses. It involves the physical facility and the people on staff. Your reputation, on the other hand, is what the members tell their friends about your club. Do they recommend you to others, or do they say negative things about you? Is your reputation based on long-term quality service to members, or are you the one who is more interested in churn selling? It's not important what you think about your club. It's more important what members and prospects think about your club and what they tell their friends.

> **Make sure you keep the promises you make in your advertising.**

First Purchase Conditions

First purchase conditions refer to the initial reasons people join your club. Why do they buy from you and not your competitor down the street? What are their visible and hidden needs that motivated them to purchase this membership? How will you find out these needs? The simple answer is to ask and listen. Find out what drives individual members into joining and then coming on a regular basis. Their first purchase conditions may vary over time, but you must attend to them at the outset.

Here are some of the first purchase conditions you are familiar with:

- Losing weight
- Feeling better

- Looking better
- Firming up
- Being close to home or work

Here are some you may not be aware of:

- Baby-sitting (for free)
- Personal training
- Spa services
- Significant other
- Self-confidence, self-esteem, self-worth (and other psychological reasons)

You can probably come up with many more. The point of these brief lists is to help you identify the communicated reasons that people will join your club. They may not be the real or main reasons, but they are the first purchase conditions. Once you know these, you must find out exactly what the new member expects from you based on these conditions.

Price/Value Perceptions

Price/value perceptions are the major obstacles every business and salesperson must overcome. Price is the most frequent objection to any purchase, and it is often a major barrier to customer acquisition. It's your job, and that of your sales staff, to make sure that the price objection never comes up. The way to do this is to build up the value of the membership. When you fully understand a person's first purchase conditions, you can focus your membership presentation on how you will meet and satisfy those conditions. Price is only an issue when the buyer does not readily see the value in the purchase.

Suppose you were planning a vacation, and you had six months to complete your planning. You call the airlines and ask for the best price. You have a great deal of time, and you would never expect to pay a premium for the flight with this type of lead time. The ticket is of very little value to you at this point, but suppose you get a call that says you must be in another city by the next day for an important business meeting. You hurry to call the airlines, and they give you a much higher ticket price than if you booked weeks or months in advance. You don't argue or negotiate because you have to get to your destination. The ticket is of great value to you, and the price does not matter.

Here's another example from our industry. We have preached the gospel for years about the cardiovascular benefits of exercise. We now have the Surgeon General's report on our side. But neither of these actions have driven people into our clubs in droves. These people still don't see the value in giving up their hard-earned money for a membership in a health club. But wait until one of them has a heart attack or gets a strong admonition from a doctor to "exercise or die." Then, you'll see them flock to the clubs in those droves you wanted. Now the value of the membership far exceeds the price or cost of it. That's your job for member acquisition and retention: Always create more perceived value beyond the cost of the membership. One way to do this is to tap into the person's emotional need state.

Need State

The need state is different from the first purchase conditions, although a relationship between the two definitely exists. While the first purchase conditions can be physical, the need state is always emotional or psychological. The overlap occurs when we talk about self-esteem or self-confidence, as an example.

You can find out members' need state or states simply by asking. You can also learn more about members by listening and looking. Listen for changes in their voices. They may speak more rapidly, raise their voices, or get excited when they hit on a need state. This change will occur whether the need state is conscious or subconscious. The same will be true for their physiological changes. When they are emotionally involved with what they are saying,

> *Treat members as individuals, focus on their needs and wants, and work with them to help them achieve their goals.*

watch their eyes, their hands, and their overall body language. You will see a noticeable change.

Get them talking about that need state. Show them you care about how they feel and their emotional reasons for joining your club. Remember that people buy on emotion and justify on logic. To keep that positive emotion going, and to build the basis for a relationship with members, pay attention to what they need. Ask for as much information as they are willing to communicate. Let them know you'll be there when they need you. Your potential for a long-term relationship with a member is based on how well you do during the acquisition stage.

Relationship Basis

This concept is really very simple. Every person joins a club with some preconceived notions of the type of relationship he or she wants with the club, its staff, other members, and friends who have also joined. It's up to you to find out what makes a good relationship for each member. Some people want staff hovering around them to make sure they are doing everything right, or they may just want the appearance of attention. Others feel that a good relationship is based on being left alone, but knowing the staff is available when needed.

Find out during the initial membership purchase what the basis is for establishing a relationship with each member, then give the members what they want. Think about when you were dating someone you liked. You did everything in your power to learn about this person, to find out what made him or her tick, and to discover why that person was different from other people you previously dated. You learned all you could about the person's likes and dislikes, what the person wanted in a relationship, and what the person would do to continue getting it. Selling a membership is the same thing, and it requires the same amount of investment and trust on your part. Each time that someone new joins your club, think of it as courting someone new.

For larger clubs, treating each member individually may seem like an insurmountable obstacle and a daunting task. But you'll find that when you do treat each member individually, you'll have fewer complaints from and longer retention of those members at lower costs, which eventually translates into increased profitability.

Post-Purchase Reassurance

You know about this concept, although you may not call it post-purchase reassurance. This is why we give people 72 hours to reconsider their membership purchase after they join. People go into a psychological state called cognitive dissonance after they make a fairly large purchase. Everyone does it, including you and me. Think about the last time you bought a car or a computer system. You couldn't wait to show it off to everybody. You wanted their opinion and/or approval of your purchase. You need their verification and justification that you made the right buying decision. This verification is how human beings attempt to resolve cognitive dissonance.

Post-purchase reassurance is a simple act on your part that tells members that they made the right decision to join your club. It involves a few simple steps. First, when members join, reinforce their decision right on the spot. Then after they have gone, call their home or office and repeat your belief that they made an excellent decision to join your club. Send them a written thank-you note immediately. This type of behavioral response compression (three follow-up activities in a short period of time) will ease any cognitive dissonance new members may have.

During these post-purchase reassurance activities, remind members of why they joined and how you will help them achieve their goals, satisfy their needs, and maximize their first purchase conditions. Let them know that you will be there for them. Of course, from a service perspective, when you make these promises, you must keep them.

In a nutshell, post-purchase reassurance has done more for more businesses in more industries to keep customers happy and save sales than almost anything else. It plays to the psychological and emotional nature of the purchase, as well as the logical side of it. You let customers know they made a wise and good decision by buying from you, and you reinforce their decision. You satisfy both sides of their brain with this technique.

Guarantee/Warranty

A guarantee can set you apart from the entire health club and fitness industry. You're already familiar with the concept of guarantees from your equipment purchases. When you buy equipment, you expect it to work without any problems for a certain amount of time. The equipment manufacturers guarantee the equipment to be free from defects in workmanship for one, three, or five years. If they have to do repair work, they warranty that work for another period of time. The same thing happens when you buy a car. You receive a warranty for miles or years of operation. Many times, your decision to buy something is based on the guarantee or warranty the seller offers.

You can implement powerful guarantees in your club beyond the three-day cooling-off period following a membership purchase. You can extend this period to 30 days. If members decide that they are not happy within the first 30 days of their membership, you refund their money and let them out of their contract (if there is one). Or you can extend this period to six months or even a year. Before you think I'm crazy, realize that the majority of your members are honest and will deal with you fairly. A few will take advantage of your guarantee, just like they would in any business. But you must operate your club for the benefit of the 95 to 98 percent of the members who are honest, rather than the 2 to 5 percent of members who will abuse your guarantee.

You can also give guarantees with your specialty programs. For example, you offer a 12-week weight-loss program, and you guarantee that participants will lose between 12 and 36 pounds during that time. If they don't lose that amount of weight, you'll refund their money or re-enroll them in the program. You only have to stipulate that they follow all aspects of the program and record their activities. This personal tracking is usually enough to ensure that they will comply with the required behaviors. If a few of them cheat you or beat you, give them their money back or re-enroll them. You'd rather have them talking nicely about you or being quiet than running around complaining to other members that you didn't live up to your guarantee.

Costs Associated With the Acquisition Phase

There are three sets of costs you must be aware of during this phase of the process. The first is the total cost of acquiring a new member. Acquisition costs are the sum of marketing and advertising costs, sales costs, cost of products used to make the sale, overhead, and salaries. All these costs figure in to how much it costs to acquire a new member. Most clubs, if they even calculate this figure, just take into consideration the marketing, advertising, and selling costs. However, to get a more accurate picture of your investment per member, I recommend that you include all these figures in the calculation.

Lost opportunity costs are those potential revenue dollars that you lose because you either didn't get that new member, or you signed him or her up and then let him or her get away. The member rescinded his or her membership during the three-day period or for one reason or another. One way to calculate these costs is to determine the average total expenditure for a member who has been with your club for one year, three years, and more than five years. If you're a new club, use whatever figures are available. Then, average those revenues and use them to calculate the lost opportunity revenues or costs to your club because you didn't keep or sign a member.

The cost of poor service is calculated based on how many potential members you lose and how many current members you lost, multiplied by the acquisition costs. In other words, how many members and how much money are you losing because your service levels are not where they should be? In some clubs, this number can be staggering.

The Retention Phase

During the Retention phase of the member life cycle, you do everything in your power to serve, satisfy, and keep your members. If you go back to the old philosophy of health club operations, the key to survival and success was a constant influx of new members. Clubs had to continuously sell memberships to keep their doors open. This constant selling created the public perception of churn in our industry. Clubs were more interested in selling to new members than they were in servicing current members.

This perception was proven, in the minds of the public, by the constant change and variety of membership sales incentives and initiatives. It was more than a program of the month. It looked like a program of the week. There were 2-for-1 sales, no payments until next year, a waiver of the initiation fee, and who knows what else. All these incentives were focused on bringing new members in the door. Even when a sale was going on, clubs didn't offer the same prices to their renewing members. Think of the uproar that created in the minds of the members, and think of it in light of today's service mind-set.

More than 10 years ago, I warned the industry at an IHRSA (International Health, Racquet and Sportsclub Association) presentation that it must focus on membership retention. IHRSA came out with a publication called "Closing the Back Door" around the same time. Yet it's taken over a decade for the industry to marshal its resources and decide that retention is a critical issue for its success. Now the presentations I give on membership retention are standing room only as club owners and managers look for the best ways to decrease their attrition rates.

The industry average for attrition hovers around 40 percent. When I interview club owners and managers, I get figures that range from as low as 8 percent to as high as 82 percent. Both of these numbers scare me because how can one club be doing so many things right to keep most of their members and another be doing so many things wrong to lose so many members each year? The important thing now is that we must all work together to figure out ways to retain our members.

As I've said before in this book, in my speeches, and in other articles, membership retention is not primarily about programs any more. It's about a business approach to serving and satisfying the members on a daily basis. Although special programs may work at times, their impact is short-lived. Retention incentive programs have the same effect as other types of incentive programs. There is a boost in the effect you're trying to create over a short period of time, and then things return to normal, whatever normal is.

Your retention efforts must focus on retention as a business. Although incentive programs that offer rewards and recognition are one activity during the Retention phase of the process, you must also concentrate on the other six activities. These activities are establishing your club's service philosophy and approaches to service delivery, conducting a gap analysis of your service offerings and the perceptions of the members receiving the services, managing the expectations of the members, managing and resolving complaints, recovering from service mistakes, and improving the satisfaction levels of your members. The following sections describe these seven retention-related activities for the member relationship management process.

Service Philosophy and Delivery

Many clubs and businesses in other industries do not have a formal service philosophy statement. Your service philosophy statement is not your mission statement or vision statement. It is a separate statement of how you plan to work with and serve your customers. It is as important as all the other strategic statements you may develop, and in some cases, it is more important because it affects the daily operation of your club.

When I ask club owners about their service philosophies, many tell me that they do whatever it takes to satisfy the members. That's a start, but it is not good enough as a philosophy statement. You need to create a statement that not only tells your members what you will do for them, but that also guides your staff in the delivery of that service. After all, how can your staff members deliver great member service if they don't know how you want them to deliver it?

No one can tell you exactly what your service philosophy should be. Only you can determine the final version. Of course, you can have other people help and guide you in its development. As the president and owner of a consulting and training firm, here is the service philosophy I've developed. Use it as a guide if you'd like. It has served me well for many years, and it lets my clients know exactly how the company will work with them:

"It is the service philosophy of Gerson Goodson, Inc. to be available, adaptable, flexible, and responsive to the needs, wants, and expectations of our clients. We achieve this by listening to them, by asking for feedback, and then by making any necessary changes to our policies, procedures, and performances based on their suggestions. We do the work for our clients right the first time and do what we can to exceed their expectations, satisfy them as customers, and retain them as loyal clients. While the client may not always be right, we never forget that the client is always the client."

This philosophy keeps the company employees committed to our customers and guides us in how we serve them. Feel free to adapt it to your club if you don't already have a service philosophy statement. Once you develop one, make sure all your employees know what it is, what you expect of them, and how you expect them to serve your members.

Gap Analysis and Closure

Gap closure is a critical issue regarding member retention. Several gaps can develop as you try to serve your members, and it is important for you to identify them so that you may close them. For example, you may run into one or all of these gaps:

1. The gap between the level and quality of service you think your club is providing and the level and quality of service the member perceives he or she is receiving

2. The gap between the level and quality of service you think is being provided and what your staff is actually providing

3. The gap between the expectations of the members and the capabilities of your staff to meet and exceed those service expectations

Once you identify the existence of these gaps, and others, you must work hard to close them. The two most important things you can do to close the gaps that may exist are to talk with your members and get them to tell you their perceptions of your service levels and quality. Have them describe their psychological and physical responses to your service. After you have this information, you can then develop and implement training programs for your employees to improve their service performance so that they can meet and exceed the expectations of members.

Expectancy Management

When what you think you're providing in the way of service differs from what the members perceive they are receiving, you will have a retention problem. People want value for the dollars, and they determine that value emotionally and psychologically by whether their expectations have been met. You must manage those expectations to stay at a level that your staff can meet with their service performance.

Expectancy management comes into play in a club setting in many ways. For example, a person joins a club and is told that there is a trained and certified fitness professional on the workout floor at all times. Then for one reason or another, be it staffing issues or other members requiring service, this member comes in, and no one is on the floor. You set a level for this person's expectations, and you've already failed to meet it.

Another real-world example is when members are promised that aerobics classes will never be overcrowded or canceled for any reason. Then one or the other situation occurs; the club puts too many people in the room or doesn't have an instructor. Again, the club failed to meet the member's expectations.

You promise the members that there will always be soap and towels in the locker rooms. Yet on some occasions, you run out of one or the other. It happens to be on just such an occasion that a member does not bring his or her own towel and becomes upset. You failed to meet that member's expectations.

Expectancy management is a very simple process. First, you have to know exactly what you and your staff can deliver in the way of customer service to your members. Then you make promises or commitments to deliver that type and level of service. You can underpromise and overdeliver, which may create a wow response from your members. But if you underpromise too often or your promises are too low-level, your members will start to believe that you're just trying to put something over on them. Although underpromising appropriately and then overdelivering wows members, you are better off making accurate promises and then living up to them. Keeping your promises will create a bond of trust between your members and your club, and that bond will help retain them.

If you fail to meet member expectations, you must solicit feedback from the members. Find out where the expectancy gap exists, why it exists, and what you must do to close it. The more you can meet and exceed members' expectations, the more they will be satisfied with your club and want to stay with you.

Complaint Management

I spent a great deal of time in chapter 6 covering complaint management. The important point to remember related to member retention is that when you resolve a member's complaint to his or her satisfaction, that member is likely to stay with you. When you resolve the complaint quickly, members are very motivated to do three things: keep their membership with you, buy something else from you, and make referrals to you. Plus, you elevate your trust bank in their minds, and they will allow you more leeway if you happen to make a mistake while servicing them in the future.

Make certain that you train your staff in the procedures for positively handling and resolving complaints. Customers who complain in any business are providing you with valuable information, plus they may become your most loyal customers if you take good care of them. Remember what I said earlier in chapter 6: You must actively solicit complaints because most people don't complain. You need the feedback and information to make improvements in your club operations and your service to the members. Instead of trying to avoid complaints or not wanting to hear them, realize that an effective complaint management program goes a long way toward member retention.

Service Recovery

I talked about the service recovery process at length in chapter 6. Service recovery involves fixing whatever goes wrong. If a member complains or is angry, or if you just blew it on some aspect of service, your recovery process will determine how much effort the members will put in to staying with you over time.

Make members feel good when you go through service recovery. Let them know exactly what you're going to do for them and by when (expectancy management), and then do it. Make sure you follow up to ensure their total and complete satisfaction. When they are satisfied, ask them what else you can do.

Incentive Programs: Reward and Recognition

Everyone likes to be recognized for their achievements. One of the basic psychological needs is to be affirmed by others. Most clubs do a good job of reward and recognition programs for their members. They give out caps, T-shirts, gym bags, workout towels, and so on. These items are very good as incentives for certain accomplishments. Other recognition devices include putting the names of members on a bulletin board for their accomplishments, extending their membership because of a certain number of referrals, and giving them gift certificates or travel bonuses for something they have accomplished.

The key here is to tie the incentive program to the performance and make sure the incentive has a high-perceived value in the mind of the member. Also, you must be aware that members of different age groups value certain incentives differently. For example, if you were going to give away a choice of a five-star spa vacation or an outdoor adventure vacation to the member who brought in the most new members in a year, you'll probably find that the baby boomers would choose the spa trip and the Generation X members would choose the outdoor vacation. The point here is to make you aware that you must select your incentives based on the person or persons who will receive the reward. Don't arbitrarily assume that everyone will like everything equally.

After you decide on your programs and the behaviors that are necessary for earning a reward, you may also want to consider a tiered reward or recognition program. This kind of program requires members to reach certain levels of achievement to receive a reward that is commensurate with that achievement. You see examples of this kind of program with frequent flier programs for the airlines and frequent rental programs for car rental companies. Try to adapt this tiered concept to your club.

Satisfaction Ratings

The last part of this phase of the process involves determining the satisfaction levels of your members. Many clubs are already involved in conducting satisfaction surveys. They hand out comment cards or longer questionnaires to determine how well they are serving the members and how satisfied the members are with that service. This is an important first step. You must conduct these surveys before you can work on member service improvements. How often you conduct the surveys is up to you, but I strongly urge you to conduct them at least quarterly. You may want to do a short survey every quarter and then an extensive member satisfaction survey once a year.

The surveys provide important feedback to you about your club operations, your staff performance, and your member services. Now it's up to you to do something with that feedback. Make the improvements suggested by the members. Find out why some of your members are only satisfied while others are extremely satisfied. Learn why any of your members are dissatisfied. Then work to improve everything.

Let's say your survey reveals that 60 percent of your members are satisfied (rated your club a 4 out of 5) and 20 percent are very satisfied (rated you a 5 out of 5). Most club owners would say that 80 percent of their members are satisfied with the programs and services received at the club. These same owners would then go after the 20 percent of members who rated the club in the lower categories and try to institute programs and services to increase their satisfaction levels, but this strategy is a mistake!

Research in the general business environment indicates that customers who rate their satisfaction as 1, 2, or 3 on a scale of 5 will demand more attention, energy, and financial resources than they are worth to move them to a higher satisfaction level. These customers have very little intent to continue to do business with their suppliers or refer new customers to them over time.

Why would you spend money on a marketing and service effort that is designed to move dissatisfied customers to higher satisfaction levels if you know they won't get there anyway? Why not spend your time and money on those customers who are more likely to do more business with you over time? In the next chapter, I'll talk more about this situation and how it affects your club's profitability. For now, think about focusing on those members who rate you a 4 or 5 and working to keep them satisfied and loyal.

Costs Associated With the Retention Phase

There are three major cost factors associated with the Retention phase. The first is the complaint costs. These are the costs you must expend to manage and resolve complaints to the member's satisfaction. These costs can involve invoking your guarantees, returns on merchandise, employee time, membership extensions to satisfy a complaint, and the cost of providing the service.

The second cost factor is the problem costs. These costs refer to the negative publicity or word-of-mouth you may receive from a dissatisfied member, and the time, money, and effort you must expend to combat this negative image. Problem costs also include the money you spend on collection efforts when members don't pay on time or when they leave without completing their payment obligations. Some businesses even include the cost of retention programs in this category.

The last cost factor of this phase is the incentive program costs. Whatever you're planning on doing to reward the members for their loyal behavior carries a cost with it. This cost eats into your profit margins, so you must be able to cost out the gifts and prizes, the staff time, and the program administration costs.

The Extension Phase

The last phase of the process is the Extension phase. This phase deals with increasing the loyalty of your members and extending the relationship with them. When I talk about extending the relationship, I'm talking about extending it over time, increasing the financial relationship between the member and your club, and increasing the psychological/emotional bond between the member and the club. All these things strongly affect how long the member stays loyal to you and your club.

As I mentioned previously in the book, and in my other books and speeches, it is imperative that club owners focus on increasing the strength of the psychological relationship with their members. You must create that emotional bond. When the costs of switching to another club are greater psychologically than the financial incentives to switch, the member will stay with you regardless of price. You get this effect through providing great service, treating the member as an individual, and working to upgrade all the offerings of your club.

This phase of the process focuses more on calculations that a club owner must make rather than activities. You have already engaged in all the activities that will improve your service, retain your members, and begin to build loyalty. Now you must learn and use the loyalty or retention calculations to continue to grow your club business and increase profitability.

Retention Rate

The retention rate is a very easy calculation. It is the exact opposite of your club's defection rate, which you know as attrition. I will make a slight distinction for you in the next section between defection and attrition, but for now you should know that the retention rate is equal to 1 ÷ defection rate. In other terms, your retention rate is the percentage of members who stay with you over a period of time.

Many clubs calculate their retention rate on a yearly basis. At a minimum, you need this number. My recommendation is to calculate it on a monthly basis and roll it up quarterly. Then, you can see trends in your membership fluctuations and determine whether these are caused by seasonality, service provision, or staff performance in some area. Because many clubs are now starting to focus more and more on retention programs and methods, and because that is the entire purpose of this book, it is essential for you to know both the exact number of members you retain over a period of time and the percentage of your membership that is retained.

Defection Rate

The defection rate is simply your attrition rate or what is left over after you calculate retention. To make a slight distinction, you may want to look at attrition as all the members who leave your club over a period of time, and defection would be the percentage or number of members who leave and join another club. If you use this fine distinction, you will have to do a great deal of follow-up research to find out who joined another club and why. This effort may not be practical or financially feasible for your club right now, based on staffing or other issues, but I can assure you that this information will be invaluable to your future success.

Although club owners say they are focusing on retention, they are actually asking and talking about what they can do to decrease their attrition rates. I strongly recommend that you start talking in terms of increasing your retention rates rather than decreasing your attrition rates. Psychologically, this change to the more positive statements has a very powerful effect on the performance and attitudes of your staff.

Defection Patterns

In addition to calculating the retention and defection rates, you must find out why people are leaving your club. People defect or let their membership lapse for a variety of reasons. It would be presumptuous of me or any club owner to assume what that reason or reasons were. You must ask former members why they left you and what you can do to win them back.

As you collect more of this data, you'll see patterns emerging related to member defections. Some of the categories or patterns that may occur may be related to the time of year the members leave (if it's renewal time, you must step up your efforts here), lack of equipment, staff performance, service level, value for their membership dollar, moving away, changing jobs, and so on. If the patterns that emerge are in your control, then you must work to change the circumstances that are leading to member defections.

This principle holds true both in and out of the fitness industry. You must know how many customers are staying, how many are leaving, and specifically, why they are leaving. Then, you can implement programs, policies, and procedures to begin retaining more members and customers.

Tenure/Half-Life of a Membership Class

This interesting calculation is rarely done. However, if you calculate tenure and half-life, you will find some interesting data that will help you improve your service and retention efforts to new members who fit into these classes. A membership class is a group of members who join within a certain time period, say a month or a quarter. The tenure of that class is how long all of them stay as members. The half-life of that class is how long it takes for 50 percent of those people to defect or let their membership lapse.

The reason this information is so instructive is three-fold. First, you can determine the demographics, psychographics, and sociographics of each class and apply these to future classes. When others join with these similar characteristics, you can predict with some degree of certainty how long they will stay with you. This information also helps you with sales forecasting and revenue projections.

The second reason this information helps you is that you can immediately identify future needs of similar people when they join. Then you can work to develop retention efforts to meet those needs early on, sometimes before these needs become known to the member. You will then create a wow factor for the members because they will not understand how you could know what they want before they even know.

The third reason for knowing the tenure or half-life of a membership class is that you can track your historical efforts and successes with trying to retain those members. If you know certain members will defect at a specific period of time, and your efforts to retain similar members of a previous class have failed, then you can limit or tone down your efforts to similar people in this new membership class. On the other hand, if certain retention activities have worked with previous class members, you can increase those efforts at the proper time.

Some businesses use their computer system to flag when a customer's class half-life is coming up. Then, the business steps up its efforts to retain that customer. It is like a combination of an early warning system and an intervention program. The key is to know who is going to leave and approximately when and probably why. Combine this tenure/half-life calculation with the defection pattern analysis, and you'll have your answers.

Lifetime Value and Average Net Worth

I talked about these concepts earlier in the book, so I won't spend a great deal of time on them here. To calculate gross lifetime value (LTV), take the amount of money a member spends with you in a year and multiply it by the highest number of years a member has maintained his or her membership (use 5 or 10 if you run a newer club). Let's say that a typical member spends $700 a year with your club between membership fees, retail and food purchases, and specialty programs. The longest any member has been with you is 10 years. Simple multiplication tells us that the LTV of a new member should be $7,000.

My question to you is what level of service are you going to provide to that member? Will it be minimal, or will it be worth $7,000 or more? Remember that if you lose this member after just one year, you are losing a potential $6,300 in revenues. As you'll learn in the next chapter, most of that lost revenue is profit.

The average net worth (ANW) of a member is the lifetime value minus all the costs associated with servicing that member. After you calculate your acquisition costs, your complaint costs per member, and your other problem costs, subtract them from the LTV to get your ANW. This number is the ANW over a one-year period. Let's say that the ANW is only $400 instead of the LTV of $700. Still, over a 10-year period, the ANW of a member is $4,000. Again, as time goes on, most of that money is profit.

There are more sophisticated methods than these to calculate LTV and ANW. They are beyond the scope of this book, and frankly, they are not necessary at this time. All you need are these two methods, and you'll have a great deal of information that you'll be able to use to extend your customers' memberships.

Repurchase Rate

Repurchase rate refers to how often members buy something from you. This something can be products, food, additional memberships, or anything else you sell. Your computer system should be able to track who buys what, when they buy it, and then how often they buy anything from you. An ideal report would include how much they spend along with how many times they buy a certain category from you.

This repurchase rate concept leads us to RFM, which stands for recency, frequency, and money. Recency refers to how close to today's date a member bought something from you. When you're trying to extend a member's loyalty, and you want to increase the frequency of their purchases (how often they buy), you should know that the most recent buyers of something are the

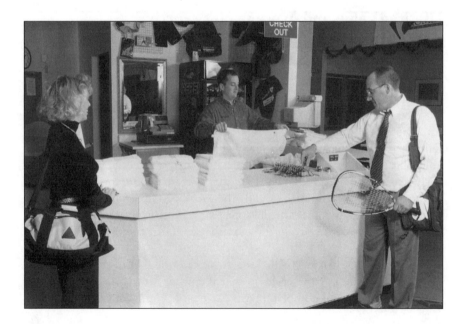

most likely to buy again. So focus your frequency efforts on your most recent purchasers.

Money refers to how much a member spent with you on each purchase visit. Because clubs have so many different things to sell a member besides memberships, they should definitely break down the purchase categories. The purchase categories will help them with their loyalty marketing programs and their entire customer relationship management program because their efforts can now be specifically targeted to each individual member.

Referral Rate

This simple calculation refers to how many members come to you through referrals versus other marketing or advertising methods. A more precise calculation of referral rate would focus on each individual member or a membership class. This calculation may give you insight and information into the characteristics and backgrounds of the referral sources, and you can again tailor marketing programs to these specific groups to further stimulate their referral behavior.

These calculations may seem like a lot to do on top of everything you're already doing to operate your club. Many of these numbers can be generated by your computer system's report mechanisms, which will make your life infinitely easier. Some of them must be done by hand, but they are still important.

When I work with clubs that are not inclined to determine these numbers and identify the defection patterns, I show them the amount and value of the information and how it helps them with future membership retention efforts. If you, for any reason, don't see the value in making these calculations and then using them to operate your club, call me at 888-2DR-RICH, and we'll talk about it. Remember that I said retention, not programming, is about the business of your success,. These numbers strongly influence your success in the club business.

Costs Associated With the Extension (Loyalty) Phase

The three major costs associated with the Extension phase are the defection costs, the customer or member save costs, and the relationship costs. The defection costs refer to the amount of revenue you lose when your members defect. This amount is different from the lost opportunity revenue calculation in the Acquisition phase, which refers to potential lost revenue from members who could have been acquired. Defection costs refer to lost revenues from members you have but lose.

Customer save costs are the monies you invest to prevent a member from leaving. They include additional marketing efforts, increased service efforts, extra incentives, and anything else you may do to save a member. Relationship costs are those costs associated with your loyalty marketing and service efforts that are designed to build up the relationship with a member. If you send out birthday and holiday cards, these help to make up your relationship costs. If you have someone on the phone calling new members to make sure they are happy, the salaries and benefits and phone fees are part of your relationship costs. Time spent in meeting with members can also be included in these costs.

There you have it—a comprehensive description of the member relationship management process as it relates to your members' life cycles with your club. All members go through each of these four phases before they decide to let their membership lapse. You will cycle back and forth between the retention and extension phases as you work to increase your retention rates and loyalty efforts. Never take any of your actions for granted or assume that your members will stay loyal. You must constantly work to keep them loyal.

The process provides you with a framework within which you can focus your marketing, advertising, sales, and service efforts. By understanding each of the four phases and the activities that occur within each phase, you can more specifically focus your efforts to what your club and members need the most. Just remember a few important things. While you are operating a business, your members are living their lives. Treat them as individuals, focus on their needs and wants before you focus on your own, and work with them to help them achieve their goals. These actions will help you improve all aspects of your member relationship management efforts.

The result of the MRM process is that you develop stronger relationships with your members; focus your marketing and sales efforts on your members' needs instead of your own; integrate all your sales, marketing, and service activities; increase both sales and service productivity; and increase member and employee loyalty. All these benefits occur just from following the member relationship management process throughout the member's life cycle with your club. That's why you must never forget that the reason you are in the club business is to serve people and help them build and live better lives. The member relationship management process helps you do the two things you want to do most: operate your club business successfully and make your members happy.

The Benefits of Retention and Loyalty

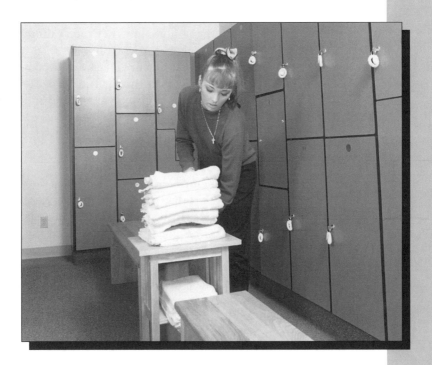

*T*hink back to the old approach that clubs used to do business. I've said this before, but it definitely bears repeating. Clubs tried to sell as many memberships as possible each month by running one special after another, regardless of how many members were leaving. It was as if they didn't care about the members they already had. Sure, they may have given lip service to current members and how important they were, but the clubs didn't do much in the way of trying to keep members for a long period of time. The prevailing mind-set was that if one member leaves, another will soon join to replace him or her.

The scary part is that, for a while, it appeared that the clubs were right. People were signing up in droves. It was like a gold rush. All of a sudden, fitness (and in the early '80s, racquetball) was in. You had to belong to the health/racquetball/fitness club. Big clubs were being built that had full-service restaurants, meeting rooms, and social areas. All this in addition to the courts, the equipment, the locker rooms, and the workout areas. It seemed that the business to be in was the health club business. That's why no one was paying attention to the members who were leaving.

I worked with one club that knew its attrition rate was 62 percent. When I asked what the club was doing to reduce it and keep members from leaving, the club managers told me they were doing nothing. They didn't think it was important to focus on because their neighborhood was still growing and people just kept joining. They figured that if a person let his or her membership lapse, no big deal. Now, the attrition rate was starting to hit them in the pocketbook, and that's why I was there. I was supposed to give them a magic bullet that would stop their defections and keep their members longer. You and I both know that there is no magic bullet. It takes a commitment to make retention work effectively.

Through some training and changes in policies, the club and I were able to reduce the attrition rate to 50 percent for a few months. But when the owners realized how much more time and effort they would have to invest in the staff and the retention programs, they decided to focus on selling new memberships rather than retaining current ones. I resigned. I wasn't going to work with anyone who wasn't committed to the importance of retention and loyalty. The club went out of business nine months after that.

If you've been reading any of the industry magazines, you know how important the topic of retention is. If you've attended any of the industry trade shows, you know that many of the presentations focus on retention. Some of them talk about programming and how to get 30 programming ideas in 30 minutes or how to develop retention motivation programs. A handful of others talk about retention as a business philosophy. You already know my opinion about the focus your club must take to stay in business and be profitable. Let me just add that you must go into the club business with the mind-set that you're going to focus on retention. When you do, the sales, revenues, and profits will take care of themselves.

This chapter is going to tie together everything you've read so far and make a strong case for you to focus your business on member retention and loyalty. I am going to draw information from other industries and make the concepts applicable to ours. I am going to provide you with many important points to consider and make suggestions on how you should revise your business approach. The benefits of retention and loyalty can be seen in people, in performance, and in profits.

You'll receive these 10 benefits and more when you take a business approach to member retention and loyalty:

1. Member retention will increase because members will be more satisfied. This increased satisfaction will also make them more loyal.

2. Your focus on retention means you're paying attention to members, which will increase their customer satisfaction. This increase in satisfaction will, in turn, increase the number of referrals each member makes to your club.

3. Your profits will increase because members will increase the frequency of their purchases from you and the dollar volume of those purchases.

4. You will naturally experience an improvement in quality throughout your club.

5. There will be an improvement in employee morale, satisfaction, and performance.

6. The more you know about your members, the more they become interdependent with you. This interdependence turns them into advocates and apostles, so they become your best sales representatives who consistently refer new members.

7. Profitability increases because member acquisition costs decrease.

8. Your defection rate decreases.

9. Loyal members will pay more for programs and services because they know they are receiving value with every purchase, plus they are committed to you.

10. Your high level of service becomes a marketing tool, a differentiating factor, and provides you with a competitive advantage.

These points should convince you about the importance of focusing on retention. If you're still not convinced, read on.

Important Points About Retention and Loyalty

You must make the focus on retention and loyalty an integral part of running your club business. You cannot, and should not, consider this focus an add-on to whatever you're doing. Retention and loyalty must be the basis for you being in business. After all, without members, you have no club. Do whatever you must to integrate the business concepts of retention and loyalty into your daily operations.

In any business, you have three groups of people you must serve, satisfy, and make loyal. They are customers, employees, and stakeholders (your investors or partners). Your success is very dependent upon signing up the right customers (members), selecting and training the right employees, and working with the right stakeholders.

What do I mean by "right"? The right members are those who join and don't abuse your system. They participate in your club activities, use the facilities, make purchases, and basically continue to be more and more profitable over time. The wrong members would be those who constantly complain for no reason (as opposed to providing you with constructive feedback), buy and return things consistently, abuse or overtax your staff, and think they can just make life miserable for everyone because they purchased a membership. The same goes for employees. Hire those people who want to work at your club, who like helping people, and who will do whatever it takes to satisfy a member. As for stakeholders, only you can determine with whom you want to be partners, sell stock to, or work closely with.

You can get all three of these important groups on your side by creating value for everyone. You can't define value; the recipient must define it. Value is a perceptual phenomenon. Your job is to find out what each of these three groups value the most and give it to them. For example, members may value extended operating hours. Regardless of the inconvenience for you, you've got to give the members what they want. You've got to open earlier and stay open later. That adds value to their membership. Having personal trainers and fitness instructors on the floor at all times also adds value in the members' minds. Allowing your employees to work out with the members adds value to both groups.

The result of any of your value-adding efforts will eventually be increased profits. A secondary benefit will be a consistent reduction in costs to operate the club and service the members. The quality of the programs and services your staff provides will naturally improve as well. Why? Because everyone is focused on providing and adding value.

This focus also helps in another way. The more the members like what they receive, the less likely they are to leave. Because adding value improves the quality of your offerings, it will also reduce the defects of your products, programs, and services. Although zero defects is a goal in total quality management, in our industry, the goal is zero defections. Zero defections means that you keep all members you should keep for as long as possible. When members move away, pass away, or have a major change in financial or social status that affects their membership, then you must expect to lose them. Aside from these reasons, your goal should be to keep them as members for as long as possible. Then, you've achieved zero defections.

The glue that holds all these efforts together is your responsiveness to customer/member needs. It is imperative that you are as responsive as a member needs you to be in order to retain that member and make him or her loyal. One aspect of responsiveness that few clubs consider, and one that is a major contributor to the success of businesses outside of the fitness industry, is the ability to customize programs, products, and services. Some clubs already do some customization when they test their members and prescribe an individualized exercise program for them.

Although it may take you a little more time to customize something than to hand a member a generic program, the payoffs to you are well worth it. There are three advantages to being responsive through customization: members are willing to pay more for a customized solution that specifically satisfies their needs and wants; members are willing to pay more because a customized solution helps them avoid other hassles and problems; and it becomes more cost-effective to customize each member's program because in the long run, that customization will motivate the member to stay with you longer. Being responsive to members has other benefits to your club. When you are responsive, you will learn more and more about members' needs. The more you know, the more you grow. You'll make fewer mistakes, and the members will be more satisfied.

Focus on retention and loyalty as an integral part of running your business.

Take a lesson from any of the five-star hotels and resorts. When you check in, they ask you a series of brief questions about your preferences. All your activities during your stay, such as requesting extra towels or pillows, are monitored. This information is fed into the computer so that on your next visit, they will know exactly how to customize their services for you. Having this information available allows the hotel to be that much more responsive to your needs.

Just for fun, I tested this responsiveness during a three-night stay at one of these five-star resorts. I asked housekeeping to make sure I had four extra bath towels each day because I worked out. It was done. I also asked them to leave the mint on the left pillow and turn the bed down only on the right side. They did that on both the second and third nights. I then asked the front desk people to provide me with a wake-up call by a person, not a recording. They also took care of that each day. They were totally responsive to my needs, so I will always be loyal to those types of hotels.

Similarly, when I work with conference and meeting planners, I prefer to speak for groups whose planners focus on my needs as a speaker. Although all meeting planners do this to varying degrees, only a handful go out of their way to make sure I'm taken care of. These planners are among the elite and the most successful in the country.

Learn from these people and adapt their approaches to your club. The more you customize your club for a member and the more responsive you are to members, the more they will reward you. How will they reward you? They will buy more from you, and they will buy more often from you. Plus, they will refer more new members to you. The result is that your club will grow because of how much you know about your members and how much you do for each one of them.

Retention and Loyalty Activities

When you take a retention and loyalty focus, you are planning for the long haul. You're more interested in getting and keeping members for life than you are in churning members to make sales numbers look good each month. If your club were mine, I'd reward my salespeople based on the number of members they get to renew more than on how many new memberships they sell. This focus on service and retention changes the mind-set of everyone working in your club. Instead of trying to constantly sell new memberships, your staff focuses on doing whatever it takes to keep your members.

One way to get your staff focused on retention is to establish various types of incentive programs for them. Base these programs on how many members they serve each month, how many they get to renew, how many they reactivate, and any other criteria you can think of related to retention. The incentives can be monetary, but they also can be other motivational items. Things such as trips, paid days off, gift certificates, and show tickets all work very well. Ask your staff members what they value as an incentive to provide excellent service and to work hard to retain members. Get a good sampling from everyone and then create the incentive program based on their input.

> *Work just as hard to keep your employees as you do to keep your members.*

This incentive program will also require that you measure their performances. Your measurements must be based on member retention, reactivation, and referrals. These are the three Rs of loyalty and business success. You should have all this data in your front desk computer system, your contact management system, or your accounting/enterprise system. Make these measurements available for everyone to see. Chart them graphically as well as numerically. Let your entire staff know how well (or poorly) they are doing with respect to member retention.

When you take this approach to operating your club, you'll attract the right people to work for you, people who enjoy working with and serving others. You can always train people to become technically proficient at their jobs in whatever field they choose. However, you cannot train people to be nice to others, to have an innate desire to serve others, and to have the motivation to help others achieve their goals. Too often in the club industry we hire warm bodies for various positions. This tactic is no longer acceptable because members want talented people who can serve and satisfy their needs. You can attract the right talent by letting everyone know exactly what is expected of them with regard to member service and retention.

One club that I worked with on their pre-opening wanted to hire a slick sales force to generate a great deal of sales prior to the actual opening. Because that is not my approach, I offered them an alternative. I suggested hiring one or two nice people who knew the industry and had previous club experience. We would focus on the service aspect of health and fitness and convince potential members that we were interested in them for the long term. We offered them the choice of month-to-month memberships or one-year contracts. There were no high-pressure sales, and we worked hard to build relationships from the start.

The pre-opening membership sales totaled 425 in 60 days. That may not be great for some clubs, but it was 225 more than the club owner had forecasted. Today, the facility is still in business, still focusing on service instead of sales churn, and has increased its membership to over 1,800. That's not to say everyone is active, but there are 1,800 paying members. Some of them have been with the club for over 10 years, and that's what is important. The service approach has led to long-term retention and member satisfaction. The revenues are generated through repurchases and referrals, which lowers the club's customer acquisition costs.

If this information sounds like a repeat of the previous chapter on the member life cycle, where I talked about lowering member acquisition costs through referrals and repurchase, then you're right. Again, I'm making a business case for you regarding the importance of member retention. Programs work and help, and I'll talk about several types of retention programs in chapter 12. But I can't emphasize enough the importance of your taking a business approach to member retention.

This approach also helps your marketing efforts. Many clubs talk about their equipment or their pricing structure in their marketing and advertising. Although you may think that this approach focuses on future members, you're wrong. This approach is strictly about your club. You need to develop a customer-focused marketing program so that members know you care about them and potential members know that, if they join your club, they will get superior service from your staff.

Member-Focused Marketing

Here are 10 things you can do to redesign your marketing efforts and make them more customer- and member-focused:

1. **Use the initial sale to stimulate a long-term relationship.** Remember the constant battle the industry has with regard to membership sales. We

are always working to overcome the public perception that we're only interested in selling as many memberships as possible in the shortest period of time and that we base our business on churn. By focusing on the relationship aspect of each sale and communicating your desire to establish a long-term relationship with every new member, you are telling that member that you are interested in them as a person.

2. **Focus your marketing on a smaller subset of potential customers who will become members.** You and your club can't be all things to all people. This recommendation requires that you specifically target your marketing efforts to reach the right customers for your club. Not every member will be profitable for you over time. By focusing on a smaller subset of the general population, you can provide those people with the marketing message they want to hear. This narrower focus enables you to more effectively spend and track your marketing dollars.

3. **Work to satisfy member needs and wants on a one-to-one basis, rather than on a mass basis.** This idea grows from the previous one. When you target a smaller subset of members, you can more easily provide those members with what they need. You can also meet and exceed their expectations. Think of this recommendation as personal training for your membership sales and service divisions. Personal trainers always focus on the individual they are working with rather than large groups, as you would have to do in an aerobics class. Run your club as if all your staff members were personal trainers of one sort or another, and their main goal is to serve and satisfy each individual member in the way he or she wants to be served and satisfied.

4. **Modify your performance, policies, and procedures based on changing member needs and feedback.** Pay attention to what your members are telling you. Look closely at your member satisfaction surveys. What worked for you in the past may not be appropriate right now. Consider how you have to change to match the changing needs and expectations of members. Make sure these changes are reflected in all your marketing materials and any communications you send to members. Let them know that you hear them and are responsive to them.

5. **Use multiple points of contact and methods of communication to consistently make a favorable impression.** This suggestion directly follows from the previous suggestion. Everyone on staff should implement your marketing efforts. Use newsletters, personal letters, flyers, posters, ads, telephone calls, and anything else you can think of to keep in touch with your members. Use these approaches to let them know you care about them and are constantly thinking of them. During your staff meetings, make sure people from every department know who your best and most profitable members are, who your most troublesome members are, and who needs a little extra

attention for whatever reason. Get everyone to learn every member's name and have your staff call members by name as often as possible.

6. **Communicate through your marketing that you want members who are satisfied and loyal and that you'll do anything and everything to help them become loyal.** This statement speaks for itself. All your marketing efforts should be focused on member retention and loyalty, and you should constantly remind your members that you'll accommodate them in any way possible. Train your staff to implement this philosophy. When you work toward member retention and loyalty, profits will naturally follow.

7. **Build rewards and incentives right into your marketing/retention efforts.** These rewards should be for both the staff and the members. Because behavior that gets rewarded gets repeated, you want to reward your staff for providing excellent member service. Plus, you want to reward your members for being great members, which they show by staying with you over time, buying from you repeatedly, and referring new members to you. You're already familiar with this concept from your member-get-a-member programs and other membership drives. Make certain you communicate the rewards people will receive for successfully participating in these programs.

8. **Know your lifetime value calculations so that you can justify more extensive member-focused marketing.** I've already told you several times in this book that most clubs don't know how much they spend to acquire a member, nor do they know their profit margin for each member. If you know these figures, then you can spend more to acquire new members, to keep current ones longer, and to provide extra value-added services to your current membership base. Clubs and companies in other industries that know the lifetime value of the customers more often than not have highly effective marketing programs that target and attract the right customers.

9. **Use customer information to stay close to the member and to improve future marketing efforts.** Collect every bit of information you can on members. Know where and when they were born, where they work, their preferred times for working out, their birthdays, the birthdays of their spouses and children, and anything else that you can learn. Use this information to keep a running dialogue and relationship going with the members. Send them birthday cards, holiday cards, tickets to their favorite shows, a gift certificate to a restaurant, or call them up just to say hello. The more information you have, the more you can target your marketing efforts. The more you target these efforts, the more your current and potential members perceive you are speaking to them as individuals.

10. **Use member-focused marketing and retention efforts to identify defection patterns.** Once you've identified defection patterns, you can work to overcome them. If people are leaving your club for one or two primary

reasons, you've got to identify these reasons and then make changes. If there are a whole host of reasons for the defections, you may need to make whole-sale changes in your people and the way your club operates. Consider your member satisfaction surveys as part of your member-focused marketing efforts and use the information you receive from these surveys. If members take the time to fill out a comment card or complete a questionnaire, they are genuinely interested in seeing you improve and succeed. Therefore, follow their recommendations and track how well they work to reduce your defection rates. The lower your defection rates, the more people are staying with you. The end result is more satisfied members who stay with you longer, spend more with you on each purchase, and buy from you more often.

TEN WAYS TO REDESIGN YOUR MARKETING EFFORTS AND MAKE THEM MORE CUSTOMER- AND MEMBER-FOCUSED:

1. Use the initial sale to stimulate a long-term relationship.

2. Focus your marketing on a smaller subset of potential customers who will become members.

3. Work to satisfy member needs and wants on a one-to-one basis, rather than on a mass basis.

4. Modify your performance, policies, and procedures based on changing member needs and feedback.

5. Use multiple points of contact and methods of communication to consistently make a favorable impression.

6. Communicate through your marketing that you want members who are satisfied and loyal and that you'll do anything and everything to help them become loyal.

7. Build rewards and incentives into your marketing/retention efforts.

8. Know your lifetime value calculations so that you can justify more extensive member-focused marketing.

9. Use customer information to stay close to the member and to improve future marketing efforts.

10. Use member-focused marketing and retention efforts to identify defection patterns.

Use these 10 suggestions to make your marketing, advertising, and public relations efforts more member-focused. Get your members involved with your marketing programs. Ask them how you can make them better and more targeted so they speak more directly to their specific needs. Listen carefully to their advice. They will tell you how to succeed. Your goal is not to sell as many new memberships as possible through these efforts. Rather, your goal is to keep as many members as possible and to build long-term, solid, and mutually beneficial relationships with your members.

Building Relationships to Increase Member Retention

We can all agree that building relationships with members and employees is what is going to make your club successful now and in the future. Although you must do everything possible to retain your members, it is just as important to keep your employees. Members don't like having to break in new employees every few months or so. Plus, when you experience a great deal of employee turnover, your staff morale and motivation decreases tremendously. So work just as hard to keep your employees as you do to keep your members.

Here are seven ways that you can build excellent member relationships. How many of them are you currently using in your daily operations, and how many of them do you have to institute?

1. **Gather accurate and current information about members and their needs, wants, expectations, likes, and dislikes.** The more you know about your members, the more you grow. It's as simple as that. After you collect this information, store it in your club database and make sure it is totally accessible to all members of your staff.

2. **Know how your products, programs, and services fit best with each member.** This is the practice of mass customization. You have the same thing that you offer to everyone, workouts, personal training, aerobics, and so on, but you customize it for each person. With members being more educated and demanding about what they want from your club and expecting more value for their dollar, you cannot operate with a one-size-fits-all mentality any longer. You must work one-on-one as much as possible.

3. **Provide value to your members with every contact.** Although it's important just to say hello to members without always trying to sell them something, they must perceive your hello as an indication that you genuinely care about them as people. When you are trying to sell them something, such as apparel or an extension on their membership, make certain

they perceive the value in what you're trying to do. Otherwise, they won't want to be bothered.

4. **Communicate regularly with members.** Keep in touch with your members. Send them newsletters, write them letters, and call them on the phone. Send them an e-mail update on what your club is doing for them. Make as many contacts as possible without becoming a pest. The more information you provide to members, the more they will feel a part of your club. This feeling will lead to commitment and loyalty on their part.

5. **Invest time to learn about members' businesses and personal lives.** This suggestion comes back to knowing as much as possible about your members. Integrate your club activities into their personal and professional lives. Make your club a part of their lives in any and every way possible. Go to where they work and live and conduct programs and seminars. Link how your fitness activities can improve all other aspects of their lives. Get to know them as well as they know themselves, and allow them to get to know you just as well.

6. **Establish a win-win partnership.** Make certain that success for both of you is dependent upon a collaborative effort. You need them to stay members for a long time so that your club can prosper. They need you to keep up with the latest in training techniques and the science of fitness so that they can continue to improve their health. Collaborate and cooperate to create an environment that works for both of you.

7. **Reward member loyalty.** When members stay with you, you should reward them in a meaningful way. That means you must first ask them what is important to them as a reward, and then give it to them. Remember that what gets rewarded gets repeated. So when a member shows their loyalty by extending their membership or bringing in new members, reward that person with something of value.

Do these seven things to build strong member relationships, and you'll find your club growing on a regular basis. Let your members know you care about them, not just as members, but as individuals. Treat them as you would someone you are seriously dating or getting engaged to. This is the peak of relationship-building. You find out about each other, you learn more about each other, you decide you want to be together, and you are enthusiastic about being together. Build your relation-

> **Make sure all your member activities focus on service and are geared to building relationships.**

ships with the ultimate result being a long-term commitment between you and the member. When you work toward this result, members want to stay with you instead of going somewhere else.

Here are 10 reasons why members will work hard to maintain a relationship with you when you've first built that relationship on a foundation of mutual trust and benefit:

1. You know how your club's programs and services benefit your members.

2. You possess an intimate knowledge of the health status of each of your members.

3. You make yourself accessible to them when they need you.

4. You inform them of new products, programs, and services and how they will benefit.

5. You help them solve their problems, both in and out of your club.

6. You are responsive to their needs and requests.

7. You follow up with them after each contact.

8. You support them in whatever they do in your club.

9. You've earned their trust so they want to refer people to your club.

10. You give them value for their purchases, so they want to continue to buy from you.

Any or all of these 10 items will increase your member retention. Your positive role model behavior will be followed by the members, and your good actions will be returned. The return will be in the form of increased commitment, retention, and loyalty on the part of your members.

Other Benefits of Long-Term Member Retention

There are some additional benefits you will receive when the majority of your members stay with you over the long term. Although a sales promotion may bring an influx of new members quickly and drop thousands of dollars to that month's revenue line, there is no guarantee that you can maintain that spike in sales. On the other hand, when your membership grows through referrals and renewals, your profitability increases because your member acquisition costs automatically decrease.

Here are five more benefits you receive when your members stay with you. First, staff productivity increases because the long-term members require less of your staff's time. Your staff can then spend more time serving newer members as well as developing new offerings. Second, employee satisfaction increases because employees get to know the members well and establish personal relationships or bonds with the long-term members. Employees are always happier serving people they know and like. Third, your market share will increase because more people will join your club just because of the high level of service you provide. They figure that if all these other members are renewing, there must be something to your service. As more people join your club, less of the market will be available for your competitors.

Fourth, you'll increase your customer share. Members will spend more money with you and at your club instead of buying the same things elsewhere. Why should members go to a sporting goods store or a department store to buy workout clothes if you have them at the club? Why should they go to a nutrition store to buy supplements if you provide them at the club? The answer is they shouldn't, and when they buy these items from you, you're increasing your customer share (also known as wallet share). Last, and certainly not least, your profitability will increase because of lower acquisition costs, as mentioned before, as well as incremental profitability from increased customer share.

I'll talk about the loyalty math concepts in the next section. For now, just realize that long-term member retention makes everything better. To tie it all together to this point, make sure all your member activities focus on service and are geared to building relationships. The relationships are what lead to long-term member retention, and retention leads to success.

The Mathematics of Retention and Loyalty

Much of the material in this section is adapted from an excellent book called *The Loyalty Effect: The Hidden Force Behind Growth, Profits, and Lasting Value* by Frederick F. Reichheld (1996). The reason I am including it in this chapter is because it is essential to your understanding of the business importance of retention and loyalty. I strongly recommend that you read this book to get more information on retention, loyalty, and business success.

Five Ways Loyal Members Are More Profitable

The five ways loyal members are more profitable boil down to common sense. Throughout this book, I've referred to them in one way or another.

1. **Base profit.** This term refers to the initial profit you make from the first sale.

2. **Revenue growth.** This ongoing revenue is generated by members who stay with you over time. Their spending tends to increase as they become more loyal.

3. **Cost savings.** The longer a member stays with you, the less you have to spend in operating costs to service that member. That's because the member starts to become self-sufficient and can do more things without the help of your staff. These savings then become profits.

4. **Referrals.** In our industry, this should be a no-brainer. The more satisfied a member is with your club, and the longer that member stays

a member, the more people he or she will refer to join. Every referral who becomes a member increases your profit on the first and subsequent sales because acquisition costs were lower. Also, you already have credibility in the new member's mind, so that person won't mind spending more with you, and these new members perceive you as someone who provides a valuable service simply because they came to you through a referral.

5. **Price premium.** Long-term members don't mind paying higher prices for increased value. As long as they get what they pay for, and then some, they will stay with you even if you increase your fees. This is the ultimate beauty of loyal members. They pay your price because of what you give them in return. If that price is higher than the club down the street, they still stay with you because the psychological switching costs are too great. When you've reached this point, pat yourself on the back. You're doing a great job.

As we're already talking about profits, here are some numbers from Reichheld's book that should interest you. When you increase your retention rate by only 5 percent, you can realize a 75 percent increase in profits over the lifetime of the member. Furthermore, a 5 percent increase in retention leads to a doubling of your membership base every 14 years. If you increase retention by 10 percent, you double your membership base in 7 years.

> *The more members like what they receive the less likely they are to leave.*

Think of the enormity of these statements. Without spending money on new member acquisition (marketing and advertising) and just focusing on serving and retaining your members, you can double your membership base in 7 to 14 years. Think of the constant profit growth this generates also. That's why I have said throughout the book that retention is a business proposition, not a program of the month. Now you have the figures to support that statement.

Retention Rate, Defection Rate, and Tenure

The industry average for member attrition (defection) is around 40 percent. At least, that's what the surveys tell us. Let's use that figure for now to calculate defection rates, retention rates, and tenure, which is the length of time a member stays with you. At a 40 percent attrition rate, the retention rate is 60 percent. Converting these rates to fractions tells us that two-fifths of our members defect every year while three-fifths stay with us.

Invert the defection fraction to get the tenure rate. A member stays with us, on the average, for 2.5 years (5 divided by 2). Although you may think you're making money off that member over that time period, you should check your costs. How much are you spending to serve and keep that member? Are you profitable with that member after only 2.5 years? If you have to replace 40 percent of your members every year, are you really profitable at all?

The picture is not all that gloomy, though. If you can increase your retention rate to 75 percent, your member tenure goes up to 4 years. Add another 5 percent to retention, meaning retention is 80 percent and defection is only 20 percent, and your tenure rate increases to 5 years. When retention becomes 90 percent, your tenure rate is 10 years, and if you can get your retention rate up to 95 percent, members will stay with you for 20 years (assuming you're open that long).

These figures are gleaned from a variety of industries and can only be extrapolated to our industry. However, they are definitely instructive and convincing regarding the importance of member retention and the contribution it makes to revenues and profitability. I suggest calculating revenue and profit figures in addition to your retention and defection rates. I know from my workshops on these topics that club owners are remiss in putting the dollars to the percentages. Whatever the reasons for it not being done before, you should now be convinced of the importance of calculating retention and loyalty rates and dollars.

Member Satisfaction and Loyalty

In a 1995 article in the *Harvard Business Review*, Jones and Sasser made a compelling argument for the relationship between satisfaction and loyalty. Again, this information is based on a variety of industries that does not include fitness, but we must learn from it.

Most clubs ask their members to complete a customer service or satisfaction survey. Without getting into the components of the survey or what is done with the results, let's talk about the responses you receive. Most surveys are answered on a five-point scale with 5 representing a high degree of satisfaction. If 3 is neither satisfied nor dissatisfied, clubs report that x percent of their members are satisfied (rated them a 4 or a 5). Yet this percentage is misleading because the 4 satisfaction rating has little or nothing to do with retention and loyalty.

Figure 11.1 shows the relationship between satisfaction and loyalty that Jones and Sasser found from their research. It is instructive to note that most clubs focus on trying to make the members who rated them a 1 or a 2 more satisfied. In reality, that is next to impossible. It is probably these members who cause you the most trouble and grief and who eat into your profits. The best thing you can do is stop trying to satisfy them and let them serve themselves or not renew. You need to focus on those members who rate you 3 or 4. Yes, 4. These are the people who are likely to switch and join another club for one reason or another.

RATING	SATISFACTION LEVEL	LOYALTY
5	Completely satisfied	Very loyal
3 or 4	Satisfied	Easily switched
1 or 2	Dissatisfied	Very disloyal

FIGURE 11.1 *How ratings relate to satisfaction and loyalty*

Looking at this figure tells you exactly where to focus your efforts. Your goal is to convert the members who rate you 3 and 4 to members who rate you 5, which means moving them from satisfied and somewhat loyal to completely satisfied and very loyal. In order to do this, ask your members what they need, want, and expect from you to make them completely satisfied and loyal. Then, give it to them. The result will be more loyal members who stay with you longer and who are more profitable.

part four

Techniques to Build Member Loyalty

CHAPTER 12

Member Retention Programs
That Work

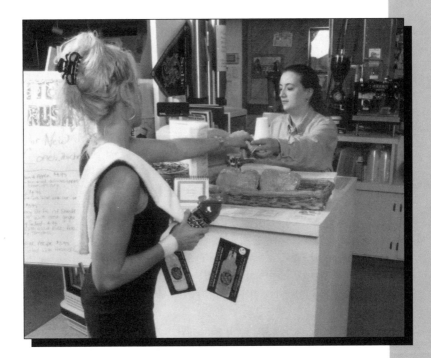

Any industry convention always has numerous presentations on retention programming. These presentations
give you ideas on what programs to implement, how to run them,
and what effect they should have on your retention efforts. Every one of these presentations that I've ever attended has good
ideas, and I recommend that you listen to these professionals. I
also want to reiterate the importance of using the programming
as a method to support your retention business efforts, not as a
replacement for them.

This chapter describes some of the programs and approaches that I've tested with clients, as well as learned from attending several presentations. Used properly, these different types of retention programs can lower your attrition rate and increase your profitability. Implementing any of these programs will help you retain your members. Combining several of these programs or running them in succession will also help you keep your members for life.

25 Member Retention Programs

Here are 25 ways you can program member retention into your club operations:

1. **Special events.** Create special events just to show members how much they mean to you. No one type of event is more successful than another. You need to use your creativity and ingenuity to develop these events and make them work.

2. **Value-added services.** The term *value-added* is getting to the point of being overused. Simply put, members must perceive that they are receiving more for their money than they expected. Some value-added services include free valet parking, free breakfast bar for early risers, free health screenings, free car wash, closed captioning on your television sets, a physician referral service, parent/child events, educational classes, and unique training seminars.

3. **Buddy system/mentors.** New members often drop out because they do not feel welcome or comfortable with the club. Assign an experienced member to be a buddy or mentor to the new member for the first month or two. You can also use a staff member in the mentor role. Whatever you do, the new member will love the personal attention and stay with you longer.

4. **New member orientation plan.** Many clubs hold a brief orientation for their new members or have a staff member teach them how to use the equipment. I'm suggesting that you develop a longer term orientation program that keeps the new member learning from a staff member over a period of weeks instead of minutes. As long as new members are gaining knowledge, they'll stay motivated. This motivation will translate into greater satisfaction and greater retention.

5. **Education classes.** Classes in health clubs are not just for health promotion anymore. Hold classes on topics of interest to your members: financial, business operations, marketing, relationships, selling, raising children, and anything else you can think of.

6. **Computerized exercise tracking.** No matter how proficient people become using computers, they still love to get their own printouts on their workouts and achievements. Like anything else, when they see their progress in writing, they tend to believe it more and they become more motivated to continue. Plus, a computerized tracking system lets members know you're interested in the technology that will help them achieve their goals.

7. **The name game.** Require your staff to learn the names of at least five new members each day. When your staff can call every member by their name, then the members will continue to stay with you because of the personal recognition they receive. Although this appears to be a very simple thing to do, and I'm sure most clubs say they do this well, you'd be surprised how few staff members know the names of a majority of the members.

8. **Touch me in the morning.** Make sure your employees touch at least five new members a day. They can physically touch them on the elbow or shoulder during a workout, or they can emotionally touch them with some motivating words. Again, I'm talking about respect and recognition, two of the most basic needs that must be satisfied for every person.

> *Make your club stand out by providing outstanding customer service to all your members.*

9. **Trust.** Establish programs and policies that show your members you trust them. These policies could relate to payments, use of towels, equipment, or anything else. The more trust you show toward members, the longer they'll stay with you. After all, why would you want to go somewhere else where you have to prove yourself to new owners and staff when your current club trusts you implicitly?

10. **Great customer service.** Do whatever it takes to serve and satisfy customers/members, and you'll be rewarded with their loyalty, commitment, and long-term membership.

11. **Change workouts to "funouts."** Make your club a fun place to be. Make workouts fun. If you can take the drudgery out of working out, you can put more members in your club for longer periods of time. Think about how many people drag themselves to work everyday. No one says they're going to have fun. Make your club a fun place to be, and you'll reap the rewards as your members reap the benefits.

12. **Instruction.** Have your staff make personal contact with each member in the club and offer encouragement plus a bit of advice on how to improve the exercises that member is performing. Members will appreciate the personal touch and will stay with you to continue to receive it.

13. **Contests.** Develop different types of contests for your members. Change the contest environment so one person doesn't always win. When more people can win a contest, more people will stay involved. Also, give out prizes that have a high perceived value, without having to be expensive.

14. **Media coverage.** Some of your members won't mind having their names in the paper or being on radio or television. Find out who these people are and make them stars of your club. They'll reward you with loyalty and long-term memberships. Additionally, when their friends see them on television or read about them in the paper, they'll probably come and join just for the chance to be a star.

15. **Empowered employees.** This could be your most valuable member retention tool and technique. Train your employees well, and then empower them to make decisions to serve the members. Next, go beyond that and provide your employees with the authority to support their responsibility of serving and satisfying the members. When employees are truly empowered, they feel better about themselves, and this feeling translates into better member service.

16. **Member feedback.** Involve your members in the club. Get them on an advisory council, solicit their feedback for club improvements, and implement their suggestions. By involving them, you provide them with an "ownership" stake, and they will stay with you longer because now they have a part in helping you succeed.

17. **At-home memberships.** Instead of letting members give up their memberships, offer them an at-home membership. This membership can range from sending a personal trainer to their home on a scheduled basis to charging them a retention fee. The retention fee is lower than their normal monthly fee, and it keeps their membership privileges active. Use this program based on the psychology that the loss of a benefit is more motivating than the gain from first receiving that benefit.

18. **Cancellation fees.** Let members know that you're so interested in keeping them for the long term that you're going to charge them a fee to cancel their membership. This fee will help them think twice about leaving you and giving up their member benefits.

19. **Zero defection.** Although the club industry defection rates vary, you can set a goal of zero percent attrition. Is this impossible to reach? I don't know. What I do know is that if you set a goal for 25 percent defection and you achieve it, you'll get complacent. It's like accepting mistakes on 25 percent of everything you do. The only way to achieve zero defection is to set it as a goal and strive for it.

20. **Recall and confirmation calls.** If your member database suggests that certain members have not been in for a while, call them, write them, or even go visit them to learn why they're not participating and enjoying the benefits of their membership. Schedule appointments for them to come in and see you personally. Offer them something for free as an inducement to come back to the club. Always remember to use your computer as a tracking, marketing, and retention tool.

21. **Clubs within the club.** Form special interest groups (SIGs) or special interest clubs. Establish cycling clubs, hiking clubs, investment clubs, and any other type of club you can think of to get members involved with each other. The more things you can provide for the members, and the more reasons they have to come to your club, the longer they'll stay with you.

22. **Summer camp.** If there is a way for you to hold a summer camp for adults and children, do it. Parents everywhere look for places to send their children when school's out. What better place than their club, where they already trust the staff? Aside from keeping members with you longer, summer camp can be a nice revenue generator for the club.

23. **Community outreach programs.** These programs are often used as a marketing tool, yet you can double their effectiveness by promoting your community services to your members. People always like to do business with companies that give something back to the community. Your outreach programs can be as simple as sponsoring a youth sports team or as complex as hosting a comprehensive health fair. Whatever you do, your in-house promotions of your work will motivate members to stay with you.

24. **Names in the news.** Most clubs have some sort of newsletter. Make sure that you put new members' names in the newsletter, as well as the names of those who refer other members to you. People love to see their names in print, and they'll continue to do just about anything to gain that recognition again. Another twist on this is that when you do put a member's name in the newsletter, send them a pasteup of the page with the masthead. They'll appreciate your extra effort.

25. **Member appreciation parties.** Show the members you care by hosting parties just for them. Let them know the purpose of the party. You can even develop a series of theme parties. Invite the members to bring guests who can then become potential future members.

Retrain to Retain

You can never stand still when training your employees. All clubs do their best when initially training their staff members to perform their duties. Now you should retrain your staff members to work as if they were five-star hotel personnel. If you want to do this quickly and inexpensively, send your staff people to any of these types of hotels, have them sit in the lobby, talk to the staff, eat in the restaurants, and observe the quality of the service. When they bring these techniques back to your club, you'll see a vast improvement in their skills as well as morale. Provide this real-world retraining as often as possible. You'll see your member and employee satisfaction soar and your member retention levels rise.

Summary Lists of Member Service and Retention Techniques

This section provides you with a variety of lists that will help you summarize all the information in the book and create powerful and effective member service programs. The information in the lists is compiled from a variety of sources over the past 10 years that I've been working in the customer service field. Feel free to copy any of the following lists, adapt them, or post them in your club. Use them in whatever way you must to make them work for you.

Most clubs just give lip service to customer service. They do just what is minimally necessary to serve their members. You can make your club stand out by providing outstanding customer service to all your members. You should also include your service techniques and promises in your marketing to attract new members. In the short run, you'll have to invest some time and money to upgrade your member service. In the long run, your investment will pay off tenfold in greater member retention, lower member acquisition costs, and improved service.

7 Steps to Successful Member Retention

1. Have a clear member service mission, vision, and philosophy. Communicate this mission to your employees, and then train and empower them to carry out your service mission.
2. Provide members with quality products, services, and care.
3. Listen closely to your members and then act on their suggestions. Do the same for your employees.
4. Pay attention to your own intuition when serving members and have your employees pay attention to their own intuitions.
5. Treat members with respect, trust, fairness, honesty, and integrity.
6. Communicate with members regularly, including current members, former members, and your competitor's members.
7. Expand your product, program, and service offerings carefully, ensuring that you can continue to provide quality member service while you grow.

10 Barriers to Effective
Member Service and Retention

1. The club and its employees have poor attitudes toward the members.
2. The club is unable to fully understand the member's current and long-term needs, wants, and expectations.
3. The club does not possess the resources to service the member properly.
4. The member service program is poorly organized.
5. The policies and procedures regarding member service are too rigid.
6. Employees do not listen and respond to members.
7. Employees do not provide members with individualized attention.
8. The club does not respond to member feedback, recommendations, and suggestions.
9. Employees and the club project a poor image.
10. Employees have too much to do with their jobs and not enough time to service the members or implement the retention programs.

From Members for Life by Richard Gerson, 1999, Champaign, IL: Human Kinetics, copyright 1999 by Richard Gerson.

The 10 Commandments of Superior Member Service and Retention

1. The member is the most important person in the club.

2. The member is not dependent on you. Rather, you are dependent upon the member. You work for the member.

3. The member is not an interruption of your work. The member is the purpose of your work.

4. The member does you a favor by visiting or calling your club. You are not doing the member a favor by serving him or her.

5. The member is as much a part of your business as anything else, including inventory, employees, and your facility. If you sold the business, the members would go with it.

6. The member is not a cold statistic. The member is a person with feelings and emotions, just like you. Treat the member better than you would want to be treated.

7. The member is not someone to argue with or to match wits with. You may win an argument, but you'll definitely lose the member.

8. It is your job to satisfy the needs, wants, and expectations of your members and, whenever possible, resolve their fears and complaints.

9. The member deserves the most attentive, courteous, and professional treatment you can provide.

10. The member is the lifeblood of your business. Always remember that without members, you would not have a business.

10 Tips for Long-Term Member Retention

1. Call each member by name.
2. Listen to what each member has to say.
3. Be concerned about each member as an individual.
4. Be courteous to each member.
5. Be responsive to the individual needs of each member.
6. Know each member's personal buying history, goals, and motivations.
7. Take sufficient time with each member.
8. Involve members in your business. Ask for their advice and suggestions.
9. Make members feel important. Pay them compliments.
10. Listen first to understand the member. Then speak so the member can understand you.

Member's Bill of Rights

The member has a right to the following:

1. Professional, courteous, and prompt service.
2. Your full and undivided attention each time the member chooses to do business with you.
3. Quality products, programs, and services.
4. Fulfillment of needs in a manner consistent with reasonable service expectations.
5. Competent, knowledgeable, and well-trained staff.
6. Attention to every detail every time he or she accesses your member service system.
7. The benefits of all your resources, teamwork, and networks to provide superior and long-term service.
8. Open channels of communication to provide feedback and voice complaints or compliments.
9. A fair and reasonable price for the products, programs, or services the member is purchasing.
10. Appreciation on the part of you and your staff for the business already given and the business that will be given in the future.

From Members for Life by Richard Gerson, 1999, Champaign, IL: Human Kinetics, copyright 1999 by Richard Gerson.

The 10 Greatest Member Service and Retention Tips of All Time

1. **Establish a unique service philosophy (USP).** Businesses need a unique service philosophy or mission statement. This USP should complement their overall business mission statement. The USP should describe exactly how members will be treated when they purchase products and services from you. The USP should also describe your preferred outcomes for every service encounter.

2. **Get member feedback.** Get member feedback any way you can. Set up member councils and focus groups, hand out surveys in your club, mail out surveys, conduct personal interviews, and beg your members for feedback. The more you involve members with your business, the more they will tell you how to improve it to satisfy them. Listen, evaluate the information, and then act on the suggestions.

3. **Use service and retention programs.** Use your member service system and your member retention program as a powerful marketing tool. Call your members, send them thank-you and holiday cards, and mail them newsletters. Do anything and everything you can to keep them informed about your business. The more your name is in front of them, the greater the probability they will continue to do business with you.

4. **Close the gap.** Quite often, a gap exists between what members expect from a club and what they receive. There is also a gap between what the club thinks members want and what the members actually want. You must constantly work to close these gaps so that your perceptions of situations are in line with those of your members.

5. **Meet and exceed expectations.** Members have certain expectations they bring to every business situation. You must meet these expectations just to satisfy the members. You must exceed these expectations to ensure their long-term loyalty. Exceeding expectations is the key to retention and repurchase.

6. **Use member reward programs.** What gets rewarded gets done. Any type of reward program aimed at the member, such as frequent buyer or referral programs, will motivate the member to continue purchasing from you. Rewards make members feel special, and they will keep coming back to the source of that special feeling. (You should also do this for your employees.)

7. **Make your public identity match members' perceived identities.** The identity you create for your business must match the perceived identity members have of themselves. This is just one factor they use in

deciding to purchase from you. The image and identity you create in the community, backed up by your actions, influence when and how long members buy from you.

8. **Perform community service and let members know about it.** Community service, charity tie-ins, and environmental issues have a large influence on member expectations for joining a club. Make sure your members know of your efforts in these areas. This knowledge will help them feel good about doing business with you.

9. **Have easily accessible, user-friendly service systems.** Make it extremely easy for members to get service from you. When they need something from you, including new products, returns, refunds, a complaint resolved, or anything else, have it ready for them. Keep your rules, regulations, policies, and procedures flexible. They should be guidelines, not laws.

10. **Train and empower your employees.** Quality employees provide quality service. Train your employees in their job tasks and in providing superior member service. Then give your employees the authority to make decisions to satisfy the member, even if those decisions go against club policy. Support your employees in all their decisions to satisfy and keep the member. After all, without members, there is no business.

From Members for Life by Richard Gerson, 1999, Champaign, IL: Human Kinetics, copyright 1999 by Richard Gerson.

One Last Thought

The success of your health club is totally dependent on how well you service your members and your employees. By now, you should have calculated the approximate lifetime value of your members. This calculation also helps you determine your individual member acquisition costs. You know what it takes to get, serve, and keep a member. You also know that your profit margins increase when you get more members to buy from you more often and to spend more on each purchase. Because the industry has a 40 percent attrition rate, you need to concentrate on member retention instead of acquisition and replacement. Your success, profitability, and longevity are dependent on how well you serve and how long you keep your members.

I'm not saying you should stop selling new memberships. I am saying you should put as much effort into your paying members as you do into acquiring new members. You definitely will be rewarded.

And, always remember that your employees are your first line of customers. These internal customers must be treated with the same care, respect, and importance as your external (buying) members. In order for your employees to provide superior service and work to keep the members, you must provide superior service to your employees and work to keep them. They, like your paying members, are the ones who keep you in business.

Finally, create the mind-set that member retention is first a business strategy and a set of programs second. Implementing various retention programs without having them tied to a sound business model is a waste of time, energy, and money. While the programs may have a short-term effect, they will not increase the longevity of your members over the long term. Build a sound retention strategy into your business model and support it with a variety of tactics. Then, your success is assured because you'll be keeping members for life.

50 Ways to Keep Your Members for Life

This book has given you numerous ideas and methods that you can use to serve, satisfy, and keep your members. Additionally, this book has provided you with techniques to go beyond customer service and retain your members. The following listing describes 50 additional things you can do to attain, maintain, and retain your members.

1. **Create a service-oriented culture.** This statement bears repeating as often as possible. You must give more than lip service to member service. Everyone in the club must be customer service–oriented. All employees must realize that they work for the member, and their job is to ensure the ultimate satisfaction of the member. Everything else is meaningless. Remember that the purpose for being in the club business, just like any other business, is to acquire and satisfy members.

2. **Have a service vision.** A vision is vital to the service success of any organization. A vision is more than just a philosophy of doing business. The vision must be the corporate cultural ethic. Everyone must believe in and live the vision in order for your club to provide excellent customer service and keep members for life.

3. **Have total support for the customer service program.** Many books recommend having top management support for a customer service and retention program. True success comes from having total support throughout the organization. Remember, although it may be top management who decides to embark on a customer service program, the staff actually implements the program. If these people do not support the initiative, then the program will not work.

4. **Put your service policies in writing.** Putting policies in writing is as much for the benefit of the members as it is for your employees. This way, there can be no mistakes or misunderstandings. Just be aware, though, that there will be exceptions to your policies, and your employees have to be able to deal with those exceptions at the time they occur. Allow your policies and employees to be flexible.

5. **Empower your employees.** This important point is another one that must be repeated. Give your employees the authority that goes with their tremendous responsibility of satisfying and keeping the member.

Allow them to make decisions on the spot to benefit the member. You then must support those decisions. Remember, their job is to satisfy the members and to keep them coming back. Employees should not have to look for you or a manager every time a member needs something out of the ordinary.

6. **Keep training your employees.** Train, train, and then retrain your employees. Give them on-the-job training, off-the-job training, tapes, books, seminars, workshops, and anything else that will help them do their jobs better. Although you may find qualified people who have just graduated from school, nothing prepares a person better for dealing with members than the training they receive on the job and in real-world situations.

7. **Market the service program.** All of your marketing should communicate the message that you provide superior member service, are interested only in total member satisfaction, and will do everything possible to keep your members. This message must be stated in everything you send out to your members, the media, and the public.

8. **Hire good and nice people.** Your employees should be good and nice in addition to being well-qualified. People who are nice to other people are usually nice people themselves. These innate people skills go a long way toward helping your staff provide superior member service and retain your members.

9. **Don't make members pay for service.** You should be willing to pay for anything related to member service, including anything the member would normally pay for in order to receive service from you. If you do not pay for the cost of service, your competition will. Then your members will become their members.

10. **Reward loyalty.** What gets rewarded gets repeated. Have you heard this before in this book? Reward loyalty on the part of both your members and your employees, and they both will stay with you a long time. Remember, although the recipient must perceive the rewards as valuable, they really do not have to cost much money.

11. **Inspect what you expect.** What gets measured gets done. Measure the service performance of your staff members, and you will see an increase in performance levels, quality, and productivity. You'll also see an increase in member satisfaction levels.

12. **Set standards of performance.** Let everyone know exactly what they must do to be considered a provider of superior member service. Make these standards as objective and measurable as possible, even though you are dealing with an intangible, service. Everybody wants to keep

score. These standards are your scorecard and scoreboard. When people achieve these stated performance levels, member retention and loyalty naturally follow.

13. **Trade jobs.** Let your employees work in other areas of the club. They will develop an appreciation for what other people in the club do. The result is that no employee will blame another one for a member problem. In fact, because the employees have experience in other areas, they will be able to solve more problems and satisfy more members without having to find help.

14. **Cross-train your employees.** This idea is an extension of number 13. Train your employees to perform other jobs. This training enables them to provide more assistance to members. It also keeps you from becoming too dependent on any one employee.

15. **Make your service systems easily accessible.** Make your customer service systems easy for the member to access. Members should be able reach a person on the telephone as soon as they call in or be able to speak with an employee who can help them as soon as they arrive at your club. Don't make it hard for members to come to you or to receive service. They will perceive this difficulty as negative and then will decide not to renew their memberships.

16. **Make your service systems user-friendly.** Members should be able to use your member service systems easily. The member is the reason for your business, not someone who stands in the way of your doing business. Make the members feel comfortable and let them know they can bring a problem to your attention or voice a complaint and get it resolved as quickly as possible. Also, let them know that they can expect to receive superb treatment during all their contacts with your club. Your member service system must be easy for the members to use, not necessarily easy on your staff.

17. **Design your service policies to be flexible.** Having written policies was mentioned previously as being important. You must have flexible and adaptable policies because each member and each situation is different. Employees must know that they can modify a written or stated policy to ensure the member's total satisfaction at any given moment.

18. **Educate the member.** You should not assume anything on the part of the member. Use every member contact as a chance to educate the member about something related to your club. Even if you are just educating them about your great personal training policy, teach them. Don't ever assume they know. They will be appreciative and will show this by continuing to renew their memberships with you.

19. **Handle complaints properly.** Use the approach outlined in chapter 6 for handling complaints. Acknowledge that the member is upset, listen carefully, assure the member you are doing everything possible at this moment to resolve his or her complaint, and then resolve the complaint. Then, when they are appreciative of your efforts, use the opportunity to increase their loyalty. Thank members for bringing the problem to your attention, apologize again for the problem, and try to sell them something else.

20. **Turn complaints into additional sales.** After you resolve a complaint, the member is most receptive to continuing to do business with you. This is a good time (and it is definitely ethical) to try to sell that member something else. In fact, such members will be appreciative of your interest in them. Sell them an extension on their membership, a wellness program, or an additional service. More often than not, they will buy from you now, and then go out and tell their friends how well and quickly you handled their problem. You will have the reputation with members of being credible, reliable, and trustworthy. Always remember that service plus satisfaction equals sales.

21. **Train your employees to do it right the first time.** This type of training will save you money and make members very happy that they do not have to return anything or complain. Repairs or additional free services are very costly. Doing it right the first time guarantees greater profitability, happier members, and more long-term members.

22. **Consider each member's lifetime value (LTV).** When a member buys from you, that is not a one-time, one-price purchase. Consider the potential that the member brings to your business. How much money could that member spend with you over a lifetime? (Remember that a lifetime in club memberships usually equates to either 5 or 10 years.) That amount is the lifetime value of a member, and that amount should be reflected in the type of service that member receives every time he or she does business with you.

23. **Beg for member feedback.** You've also heard this one before. It's not enough to send out surveys or leave comment cards at the reception desk. You must get as much member feedback as possible, even if you have to beg for it. When members are asked their opinion, and then they see you have implemented their suggestions, they will continue to do business with you, and they will recommend that friends come to you also. Do whatever you can to solicit their opinions and comments. This feedback is like getting consulting services for free.

24. **Identify member values, beliefs, and standards.** Your service programs must be geared to the values, beliefs, and standards of your members. This will tell them you're interested in them, and they will want to stay with you for longer periods of time as a result. Set up all your service programs so they are geared to and for the member rather than for your business. If a conflict exists between member values and your values, invite your members into the club for a discussion to find out why the difference exists and what can be done about it. Then decide whether you must modify your position to maintain member satisfaction and loyalty. Whatever you do, just the fact that you're considering members' values and beliefs will make the members' psychological switching costs very expensive, perceptually.

25. **Get and use employee ideas.** Your employees who have daily contact with members know more about what members need, want, and expect than you or any other manager could ever hope to know. Get feedback from your employees, listen carefully to their suggestions, and then implement as many as possible. Research shows that the best service companies not only get more ideas from their employees, they use more of them. Using employee ideas also makes employees feel wanted and cared about. Furthermore, it shows employees that you think as much of them as internal members as you do your external, dues-paying members.

26. **Be fair and consistent.** Members may not always like or agree with what you are doing for them, but as long as you treat members fairly and consistently, they will respect you for it. This fairness and consistency also enhances your credibility, which is essential for building loyalty and retaining members.

27. **Underpromise and overdeliver.** One of the ways clubs fail to satisfy and keep their members is that they overpromise and underdeliver. Overpromising establishes very high expectations on the part of the member. Usually, the club staff has difficulty reaching these expectations, and the member goes away disappointed. On the other hand, if you set realistic expectations for the member regarding your quality and level of service, and then you exceed those expectations, the member is more than satisfied. Remember, though, that you should not underpromise to such an extent that it is insulting to the members. They will see through you in a minute and take their business elsewhere.

28. **Compete on benefits, not products or prices.** Members can always find another club offering a lower price, somehow, somewhere. You must always remind your members of the benefits of doing business

with you. You can find features in every club and type of membership, but benefits are unique to the way you do business. Promote your benefits to the members on a personal level, and they will stay with you.

29. **Remember that high-touch is more important than high-tech.** High-tech equipment gets people to say, "Wow!," but it doesn't get people to care about other people. Your club needs high-touch in order to be successful. Stay close to members. Get to know each other well. The closer you are to members, the longer they will do business with you. After all, when you show you care, you become like one of the family. Members don't care how much you know about health and fitness until they know how much you care about them.

30. **Ask members what they want.** Constantly ask your members what they want from you, what you can do for them, and how you can do it better. They may want a new product, program, or service, extended hours, or just something minor that will make them happier. You will never know unless you ask. After you ask, you must give them what they want. They will reward your generosity with loyalty. Remember, ASK is an acronym for always seek knowledge.

31. **Practice daily service management.** Every employee in every department is involved in providing superior service with the ultimate goal being to keep the member for life. You should do everything possible to make everyone's job easier, and the employees should work together to make their jobs easier and to make it easy for the members to get what they want. If there is a problem during the day, make the necessary adjustments and resolve it quickly.

32. **Know the cost of losing a member.** Everyone must know the lifetime value of a member. They should also know the cost of losing even just one member and the effect it can have on your club's profitability. You can be sure that employees who are paid on an incentive basis according to how many members are retained over a certain time period will do everything possible to service and retain the members.

33. **Know your competition.** What are your competitors providing in the way of member service? What are they doing to retain their members? Are they offering more benefits, better service policies, or are they just being nicer to the members? Find out, and if they are doing something you're not doing, then just do it yourself. If it works for them, it will probably work for you.

34. **Conduct ongoing market and customer research.** You can never have enough information about your members. Do surveys, interviews, and whatever else it takes to find out what the marketplace wants. Then

adapt your club service orientation accordingly. Information is not power unless you know how to use it.

35. **Conduct internal assessments.** Constantly evaluate what your club is doing in the area of member service, satisfaction, and retention. Interview your employees, have them fill out questionnaires, ask your members at the point of purchase how you're doing, and then use this information to improve your service and retention efforts.

36. **Know what your members need, want, and expect.** Club owners and staff tend to think members need, want, or expect one thing when they really desire another. This difference causes gaps in perceptions about service delivery and quality that ultimately lead to lost members. Find out what the members need, want, and expect, and then give it to them. Close those perceptual gaps so you can retain your members.

37. **Find, nurture, and acknowledge member service champions.** Every business has one, two, or several employees who are true member champions. Find out who these people are, nurture and support them, and then make them role models for the rest of the staff. Reward their behavior in a variety of ways. Your other staff members will upgrade their service performance to this level in order to receive similar rewards. The result is a highly motivated, service-oriented staff and a group of satisfied and loyal members.

38. **Keep in mind that effective communication is critical to success.** Every problem between people is the result of poor communication. Therefore, train your people to develop effective communication skills: how to speak so others will listen, how to listen first, how to understand others before trying to be understood, how to receive and give feedback, and how to develop rapport with members.

39. **Remember that rapport is the key to successful communication.** You can acquire and use the technical skills of communication, but if there is no rapport, there is no communication. The skills of developing rapport can be taught, and your employees should learn them. When employees and members are in rapport, there is a feeling of trust and a desire to continue to do business.

40. **Smile.** Smiles are important when interacting with a member. Smiles get a smile in return, but smiles do not guarantee quality member service. Smile training is not service training. Smiles must be part of employees' daily behavior, and something they do because it makes them feel good and it makes the members feel good.

41. **Make members feel important.** You know exactly how you feel when someone pays attention to you and makes you feel important. The more

important you make members feel, the longer they will do business with you. Call them by name, ask them to tell you about themselves, and ask questions about their accomplishments. Make them feel important. Your reward will be a lifetime member.

42. **Promote your members.** That's right, your members. Use them in your marketing and promotion efforts, with their permission, of course. Let them tell their stories to other members and prospects. This third-party endorsement breeds tremendous credibility, and your members will love being involved.

43. **Create a member council.** A member council is like a board of directors or an advisory board, only it is made up of just your members. It can also serve as a focus group. The purpose of this group is to meet regularly to scrutinize your business and the service you are providing. The council makes suggestions, and you act on those suggestions. Membership in the council makes members feel as though they are part of your club operations, and this feeling breeds loyalty and long-term commitment.

44. **Market frequent referrer programs.** Establish a reward program for your frequent referrers. You can use coupons, punch cards, or anything else that helps you keep track of how often members refer new members to you. Then when they reach a certain number of referrals, you reward them with a gift of some kind. The gift can be a deep discount coupon, a free product or service, an extension on their membership, or something more expensive, such as a trip. The purpose of this type of program is to get them excited about continuing to stay a member and referring others to you.

45. **Accept only service excellence.** Expect average performance and service, and you'll get exactly that. Therefore, set your expectations of your employees high. Accept only excellent service performance, and realize you must train your staff to achieve these levels of performance. Good enough should never be good enough.

46. **Remember that employees are members, too.** Never forget this statement. Employees are your internal members, your first line of members, and each of them has a prospect they can refer somewhere in the value chain. Every employee must provide excellent member service to every other employee so that they all can provide superior service to members. This is the only way to guarantee member satisfaction and retention.

47. **Let members know you care.** Send them thank-you cards, holiday cards, and anything else you can to show them you care. Keep in

constant contact with them so they never forget your name. Teach them that whenever they need something, they can come to you for it because you care. Spend time and money marketing your caring attitude to your members.

48. **Make service results visible.** Although it is true that what gets measured and rewarded gets done, it is also true that what is visible gets improved upon. Post your member comment cards and letters for all members to see. Create a testimonial book for members to read. For employees, post their performance results in their lounge or locker room. Visibility enhances credibility, and credibility is only enhanced by improved performance. Make service results visible so that your employees will constantly improve and your members will be the beneficiaries of this improved service.

49. **Go the extra mile.** When a member wants something from you, give it to him or her. Then do something extra. This little extra will go a long way to ensure a member's loyalty. For example, when you resolve a complaint to a member's satisfaction, give the member something extra to take away with him or her from the situation. The member will be very grateful, and you will now have a long-term member.

50. **Make your marketing reflect your member service.** All of your marketing efforts should communicate your member service message. In today's competitive marketplace, the only thing that differentiates clubs from one another is the level and quality of their member service. Member service is the major criteria people use to decide whether to join that club. Remember that member service is a very effective and powerful marketing tool, and that marketing is a very effective and powerful member service tool. Combined, the two will help you keep your members for life.

Now, review everything you are doing and make it better. Whatever you're doing now to service and satisfy your members may not be sufficient to keep them tomorrow. A competitor will come up with a better membership deal at a lower price that has more benefits and superior member service. You have to stay one step ahead of your competitors. You must not only know what they are doing now and are going to do in the future, you must also be proactive in your service efforts. Review everything you're doing to provide member service, and then do whatever it takes to make it better. The result will be a large base of loyal and long-term members.

Index

A

accessibility xiii, 30-32, 48
advisory councils 141-142, 210
appearance of health clubs 45, 151
at-home memberships 192
attribute ratings 126-127
attrition. *See* defection
average net worth (ANW) 165-166

B

babysitting 39
billing accuracy 46
Bill of Rights for members 199
buddy system 190
buyer's remorse 137-140, 155

C

cancellation fees 192
CARE process 148-168. *See also*
    member
relationship management
child care 39
communication
    effective 42-43, 102-103
    frequent 26, 179-180
    importance 48, 209
    member education 205
    multiple points of contact 176-177
community service programs 193,
    201
complaints. *See* dissatisfaction
computer and technology support
    xii, 23, 34, 75-77, 191
contests 192
costs
    of lost members 13, 208
    of lost opportunities 8, 13, 59
    of member acquisition 8, 13, 59,
        150, 156, 167-168
    of member replacement 13, 59
    of member retention 162
customer satisfaction. *See* member

satisfaction
customer service
    attribute ratings 126-127
    barriers to 196
    benchmarking 125-126
    cards to members 133-134, 210-
        211
    continual improvement 26-27, 118
    free 204
    frequent buyer programs 132
    frequent referral programs 132-
        133, 210
    importance 3-18, 38, 56-60
    making it work 19-32, 41
    management committment 17,
        23, 203
    as a marketing tool 129-143
    measurement of 117-119, 204
    member perception of 4, 23, 34,
        114-116
    payoff of 7-12, 58-60
    philosophy 157-158, 197, 200
    poor 8-9, 10-12, 16-18, 59
    setting up systems 21-22
    special events 141, 190, 194
    Standards of Performance (SOPs)
        23-24, 125, 204-205
    statistics of 10-12
    superior member service 34-45
    techniques 194-201
    visibility of 211
    the wow factor 39-40
    written policy 203

D

data collection 121-127, 208-209
defection
    cancellation fees 192
    management of 62-63
    patterns 164, 177-179
    rates 52, 163-164, 170, 183-184
    reasons for 11, 50

defection *(continued)*
    responses to 130-131
    zero 193
dissatisfaction
    complaints and 34, 43
    cost of 8-9
    importance of listening 86, 89
    managing angry members 84-85,
        87-93, 95-96
    member retention and 96-97,
        160, 206
    resolution of 10, 16
    restitution 90, 95
    turning complaints into sales 91-
        97, 206
    why members are angry 83-85,
        87-91

E
education classes 190
empathy, importance of 49, 89, 95,
    107-108
employees
    attitudes 17, 24, 55, 77, 172, 204
    compensation 24-25
    as customers 16, 140-141, 210
    empowerment of xi-xii, 17, 192,
        201, 203-204
    input from 207
    job trading 205
    retention 24, 174-175, 209
    rewards for 25-26, 31, 134-135,
        177
    training 16, 20-21, 28-32, 194,
        204, 206
exercise tracking 191
expectations
    determining 37-39, 44, 114-117,
        209
    expectancy management 159-160
    meeting 36-37, 116, 200
    the wow factor 39-40
extension 52-53, 162-168

F
frequent buyer programs 132

frequent referral programs 132-133,
    210

G
gap closure 158-159, 200
guarantees 137-140, 155

L
lifetime value (LTV) 12-15, 165-
    166, 177, 206
listening 86, 89, 104-110
loyalty
    activities 174-175
    benefits 182-183
    management of 61-62
    referral rate 166-167
    repurchase rate 166
    rewards for xii, 160-161, 180,
        200, 204
    satisfaction and 184-185
    variable pricing and 63-65
The Loyalty Effect (Reichheld) 182

M
management commitment 17-18,
    23, 28-30, 203
marginal net worth 14-15
marketing
    customer contact 149-150
    expenditures for 14-15
    focused 176
    frequency 62
    member-focused 131, 175-179
    promises made xii-xiii, 116, 207
market share 10
market value pricing (MVP) 63-65
media coverage 192-193
member alliances 141-143
member contact xii, 69-71, 149-
    150. *See also* communication
member feedback xii, 192, 200, 206,
    208
member-get-a-member programs 132
member needs
    basic 35-36
    customizing 173, 176

determining xiii, 35, 44, 61-62,
114-117, 209
new members 153
member perception 34, 114-116,
152-154, 162-163, 200-201
member relationship management
(MRM)
acquisition phase 150-156
contact phase 149-150
extension phase 162-168
overview 20, 148-149
retention phase 156-162
member retention
activities 174-175
barriers to 196
benefits 170-171, 181-184
business growth by 60-65
club relationship and 179-185
complaints and 96-97, 160, 206
frequent buyer programs 132
gap closure 158-159, 200
half-life 164-165
importance 51-54, 202
member-oriented clubs 54-56
programs xiii, 189-194, 200
rates 183-184
recall and reactivation programs
135-137, 193
requirements 197, 198
techniques of 132-143, 156-162,
194-201
members
angry. *See* dissatisfaction
Bill of Rights 199
casual 148
demographics 164-165
information on 179-180, 206-
207
perfect 43-44, 172
rating by 44-50
types of 40-44, 92-93
understanding xii, 48-50, 54-55
member satisfaction
how to gain 37-39
loyalty and 184-185
measurement 113-118

ratings 123-124, 161-162
report cards 124-125
research methods 120-122
retention and 112
member service. *See* customer
service
membership referrals 132-133, 166-
167, 182-183, 210
membership renewal 52-53, 162-168
membership termination. *See*
defection
mentors 190
mission statements 28-30

N
name recognition 4, 48, 76, 101, 191
new membership 150-156, 190

O
ombudsmen 142

P
perceptual maps 126-127
phone calls. *See* telephones
post-purchase reassurance 154-155
price premium 183
profit 15, 117, 165-166, 182-184.
See also marginal net worth
promise-keeping xii-xiii, 116, 207.
See also expectations

R
rapport with members 100-104
receptionist attitude 4, 19
reliability 45-46
renewal 52-53, 162-168
repurchase rate 166
reputation of club 151
research methods 121-127, 208-209
responsiveness 46, 172-173
retention. *See* member retention
revenue management 63-65. *See also*
profit
reward and recognition programs
132-135, 160-161
risk reversal 137-140
rule of 10s 11

S

satisfaction. *See* member satisfaction
security 47
service-oriented culture xi, 31, 203.
    See also customer service
Service Quality Measurement
    System (SQMS) 123
service recovery process
    managing angry members 83-91,
       160
    steps in 94-96
    turning complaints into sales 91-
       97
smile training 20, 101, 209
special interest groups (SIGs) 193
staff. *See* employees
Standards of Performance (SOPs)
    125, 204-205
summer camp 193

T

tangibles 45
telephones
    behavior standards 71-75
    call completion 77
    confirmation calls 136-137
    developing dialogues 73-74
    initial contact 69-71
    prepaid calling cards 133

    response time 72-73, 80
    returning calls 37, 46, 78, 80
    standardized greeting 73, 80
    tips for 76-78
    tone of voice 72, 74-75
    transferring calls 76-77, 80
    wording 78-81
tenure 183-184
thank-you cards 133, 210-211
touch, importance of xii, 191
training
    employees 16, 20-21, 28-32, 194,
      204, 206
    smile 20, 101, 209
    telephone 72

U

unique service philosophy (USP)
    200

V

value-added services 39, 172, 190
vision statements 29-30, 203

W

warranties 137-140, 155
weight-loss programs 139
word of mouth 7-8, 10-13, 59-60
wow factor 39-40

About the Author

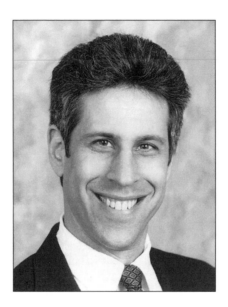

Richard F. Gerson is president of Gerson Goodson Performance Management. He has lectured extensively and conducted workshops and seminars across the nation on customer service, retention, and club business. He has been a featured speaker at many industry conventions, and he is one of the International Health, Racquet & Sportsclub Association's top speakers. He has written 10 books on marketing and customer service, including *Marketing Health/Fitness Services* and *Beyond Customer Service*.

Gerson received his PhD in Sports Psychology from Florida State University in 1978. He is certified as a management consultant, professional consultant, professional marketing consultant, and American College of Sports Medicine health/fitness director. In his free time, Gerson enjoys reading, exercising, playing basketball, and spending time with his family.